T0260946

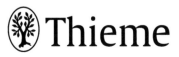

For my boys, Joshua and Joel

Visceral Manipulation in Osteopathy

Eric U. Hebgen, DO, MRO

Private Practitioner
Königswinter, Germany

213 illustrations

Thieme
Stuttgart · New York

Library of Congress Cataloging-in-Publication Data
is available from the publisher.

This book is an authorized translation of the 3rd German edition
published and copyrighted 2008 by Hippokrates Verlag, Stuttgart.
Title of the German edition: Viszeralosteopathie – Grundlagen
und Techniken.

Translator: Sabine Wilms, PhD, Taos, NM, USA

Illustrator: Christiane von Solodkoff, Neckargmünd, Germany

Important note: Medicine is an ever-changing science undergoing
continual development. Research and clinical experience are con-
tinually expanding our knowledge, in particular our knowledge of
proper treatment and drug therapy. Insofar as this book mentions
any dosage or application, readers may rest assured that the
authors, editors, and publishers have made every effort to ensure
that such references are in accordance with **the state of knowledge
at the time of production of the book.**

Nevertheless, this does not involve, imply, or express any guaran-
tee or responsibility on the part of the publishers in respect to any
dosage instructions and forms of applications stated in the book.
Every user is requested to examine carefully the manufacturers'
leaflets accompanying each drug and to check, if necessary in consultation with a physician or specialist, whether the dosage sched-
ules mentioned therein or the contraindications stated by the
manufacturers differ from the statements made in the present
book. Such examination is particularly important with drugs that
are either rarely used or have been newly released on the market.
Every dosage schedule or every form of application used is entirely
at the user's own risk and responsibility. The authors and publishers
request every user to report to the publishers any discrepancies or
inaccuracies noticed. If errors in this work are found after publication, errata will be posted at www.thieme.com on the product
description page.

MIX
Papier aus verantwor-
tungsvollen Quellen
FSC® C089473
FSC
www.fsc.org

© 2011 Georg Thieme Verlag,
Rüdigerstrasse 14, 70469 Stuttgart, Germany
http://www.thieme.de
Thieme New York, 333 Seventh Avenue,
New York, NY 10001, USA
http://www.thieme.com

Cover design: Thieme Publishing Group
Typesetting by Sommer Druck, Feuchtwangen, Germany
Printed in Germany by Beltz Grafische Betriebe

ISBN 978-3-13-147201-4   2 3 4 5 6

Foreword to the English Edition

When asked to consider writing a foreword to *Visceral Manipulation in Osteopathy* by Eric Hebgen, DO, I was conflicted but intrigued. Leaving the next day to lecture in Australia, I had hoped to empty my plateful of writing projects on the long flight, yet treatment of visceral dysfunction was near dear to my heart (*no* pun intended). In the end, the title of Chapter 3 proved impossible to resist. I offered to examine the text and happily so.

The clear, uncluttered diagrams and dynamic pictures of osteopathic manipulative technique (OMT) immediately impressed me. Coupled with the publisher's spacious layout, *Visceral Manipulation in Osteopathy* was remarkably easy to read and "digest" (pun *intended* for a cooking analogy!). The author is an effective chef who has carefully balanced precise appetizers and chosen just the right amount in each entrée to nourish—but not over-stuff—clinicians.

- **Appetizers:** In his first four chapters, the author pares down and deconstructs several key osteopathic approaches; treatments reflecting both European and American flavors. For complete recipes and their rationale, the reader should really return to the original texts; but for an overview or a quick trip down "memory-lane," the author handily summarizes terminology and many key concepts related to visceral treatment.
- **Entrées:** Having introduced ingredients (concepts and techniques) in the first four chapters, Eric Hebgen then

specifically serves up 18 additional organs in his wonderfully uncomplicated style. His simple clarity provides immense clinical practicality.

I would like to close this foreword by observing that in 1990 when we wrote our first text, *Osteopathic Considerations in Systemic Dysfunction*, we could not have imagined its impact. In later texts and editions, we continued to build upon the acknowledged work of our respected teachers and mentors (especially Korr, Denslow, Kimberly, Frymann, and Zink), just as they built upon the work of Sutherland, Chapman, Burns and others. As future texts synthesize improved, coordinated osteopathic approaches promoting health and visceral homeostasis, they will benefit from access to this text—I know our subsequent editions will.

Because of its clear explanations, quality graphics and intent to convey some of the contributions of the author's colleagues and teachers, I recommend you make this text part of your library. While it benefits from a number of practical OMT "recipes," in caring for patients I trust you will find that *Visceral Manipulation in Osteopathy* will be more than a mere cookbook.

Prof. Michael L. Kuchera, DO, FAAO
(Author of Osteopathic Principles in Practice,
Osteopathic Considerations in Systemic Dysfunction,
and Osteopathic Considerations in HEENT Disorders)

Foreword to the 3rd German Edition

During the 150 years in the history of osteopathy, numerous approaches have been developed.

Andrew Taylor Still, the founder of osteopathy, was far ahead of his times and formulated a number of thoughts that continue to enjoy unchanged validity for contemporary medicine and for osteopathy. It was his desire to warn and preserve the medicine of his times against overly radical specialization and mechanization. He advocated a holistic and individualized perspective in medicine.

For this purpose, he emphasized placing the patient at the center of the consultation. His ideal of medicine was to first do everything in one's power to activate the autoregulatory powers of the patient. It was only when the limits of autoregulation were reached that allopathy should get involved. His first yardstick for the healthy functioning of the human body was movement, in the largest sense of the word.

Eric U. Hebgen, the author of the present book, and his teacher Josi Potaznik have grasped the meaning of this philosophy. Especially in our modern world with its host of stimulations and overstimulations, the osteopathic view of the patient is gaining new significance. It offers an extremely interesting approach, in the context of the viscera in particular. The decision to write this book was therefore not far-fetched. To create a comprehensive survey, Eric U. Hebgen has adopted and integrated much information from previous publications by different authors. This book is also rooted in the visceral instructions by Dr med Josi Potaznik, DO, who has collaborated in the development of visceral instruction at the Institute for Applied Osteopathy for a long time.

The present book serves not only as a general treatment of visceral manipulation, but also as a guidepost and textbook, describing the organs according to osteopathic criteria in their physiologic movement, defining movement disorders, and presenting pathologic effects.

Werner Langer, DO
Director, Institute for Applied Osteopathy
Bitburg, Germany

Preface

It is my pleasure and honor to offer you this book, which was first published in Germany in 2003 as *Viszeralosteopathie—Grundlagen und Techniken*, now in its English translation as *Visceral Manipulation in Osteopathy*. The publication of an osteopathic book in the "mother tongue" of osteopathy, as it were, appears particularly significant to me. I hope that you will find suggestions and inspiration for your daily work.

The osteopathic manipulation of the internal organs is as old as osteopathy itself. Andrew T. Still's books show that he already treated the internal organs. He describes manipulations that primarily affect the organs through the circulatory system and aim at strengthening their self-healing powers. William A. Kuchera, DO, and Michael L. Kuchera, DO, compiled and refined these treatments in an outstanding book that was published in 1994. This traditional American treatment approach is part of this book, as is the reflex therapy according to F. Chapman, DO, an American osteopath who at the start of the twentieth century discovered the reflex points named after him and linked them to certain organs, as a result of which we know that treating the points improves the health of the organ.

European practitioners also began to manually treat the abdominal organs in the late nineteenth century. The Swedish gymnast Mårten Thure Emil Brandt (1819–1895), for example, developed a diagnostic and therapeutic method for treating the organs of the lesser pelvis. Thus, a repositioning technique for uterine prolapse is named after him, which is still used successfully today. Henri Stapfer, one of Brandt's students, further refined these methods. The French physician Frantz Glénard (1848–1920) also described visceral palpations and manipulations of different organs systematically during this time. In addition, he introduced a first visceral concept.

In the 1970s and 1980s, French osteopaths such as Jacques Weischenk, DO, in turn took on the known treatment methods and developed them further. And, finally, we have Jean-Pierre Barral, DO, to thank for the fact that the visceral manipulation of the internal organs could be established as a part of osteopathy in Europe. He systematized and structured existing information, carried out his own studies, and published a visceral concept that has become the most widespread model in European osteopathy. In the present book, I have therefore devoted the largest amount of space to Barral's therapeutic approach.

Furthermore, the two Belgian osteopaths Georges Finet, DO, and Christian Williame, DO, also carried out extensive studies in the 1980s to investigate the mobility of the organs in relation to the movements of diaphragmatic breathing. On the basis of their research, they developed a fascial treatment of the internal organs that surely deserves more attention. In this book, I introduce one part of this treatment concept that I consider the most effective.

For many people, manual treatments of the internal organs initially appear strange, and they may ask why we should even push around on the abdomen at all. Thus, we should take into consideration the fact that the internal organs are affixed mechanically to each other as well as to parts of the locomotor system and are subject to the same physical laws as the rest of the body. If we therefore recognize them as part of the mechanics of the body and take into account the anatomical connections, we can see how a disturbance in the movement of an organ has an affect on other parts of the body. Bear in mind: I am referring here to an osteopathic dysfunction, as it occurs also in the locomotor system, and not to an illness of an organ, even though in such cases Andrew T. Still himself established the circulatory treatment method. Thus, I am firmly convinced that the osteopathic manipulation of the internal organs presents an enrichment of therapeutic skills. Anybody who has personally discovered them will never want to manage without them again.

Eric U. Hebgen, DO, MRO

Introduction

Explaining the Concepts of Jean-Pierre Barral, Georges Finet and Christian Williame, William and Michael Kuchera, and Chapman

The following chapters offer a description of the osteopathic manipulation of the internal organs. I will introduce you to four treatment concepts that have one feature in common: all of them use the anatomy of the body as the foundation for the development of each particular concept. In the following paragraphs, I would like to explain the differences between these concepts.

The manipulation of the internal organs according to **Jean-Pierre Barral, DO,** is the standard method of visceral osteopathy in Europe. In this method, Barral views the organs from a mechanical perspective: organs form visceral joints with another organ or a part of the locomotor system, e.g., the diaphragm. Similar to joints in the locomotor system, the partners of a joint move against each other in fixed directions and ranges. To ensure that this movement is executed with as little friction as possible, the partners of a parietal joint are characterized by a smooth surface and by the synovium, which produces small amounts of joint fluid. Likewise, the organs have a smooth surface as their external surface is sealed off by a layer of serous skin. This layer is the peritoneum, the pleura, or the endocardium. Furthermore, we find a small amount of fluid in the serous cavities between the organs. The organs do not move against each other haphazardly but are subject to certain laws: they are fastened to each other and to the locomotor system by the mesenteries, omenta, or ligaments. This limits their range of motion. We also find this feature in the joints of the locomotor system. Ligaments permit and limit the extent and direction of movement.

Barral hence constructs his theory parallel to the parietal joints. His treatment techniques are also, to a large extent, informed by them. Similar to the parts of a joint, the organs are tested for their ability to move and directly treated to increase mobility, until a normal range of motion is restored. It is only his concept of visceral motility that follows a more energetic approach, which I will treat in more detail below.

Georges Finet, DO, and **Christian Williame, DO,** two Belgian osteopaths, carried out extensive radiograph- and ultrasound-supported studies in the 1980s, to examine the movements of the abdominal organs in relation to diaphragmatic breathing. In the course of their research, they discovered organ movements that follow certain rules. For the organs that they studied, they defined movement directions and extents, which largely concur with Barral's results. In addition, they developed a treatment method to influence disturbed organ movements and were also able to control their method using X-rays or ultrasound waves. In contrast to Barral, who palpates the organs and moves them directly in his mobilizing techniques, Finet and Williame utilize the anterior parietal peritoneum in their therapy. By moving the peritoneum, they achieve a mobilizing effect without palpating the organ itself. They call their method fascial because the peritoneum is seen as fascia and connects all abdominal organs with each other. If you pull on one part of the anterior peritoneum, this also has an effect on a distant region, e.g., the peritoneum of the pancreas. You could compare the peritoneal cover to a balloon: if you push or pull on one part of the balloon, this pull spreads throughout the entire balloon and deforms it.

Ultimately, both treatment concepts succeed in restoring the physiologic mobility of an organ, with the only difference being that Finet and Williame do so a little less invasively. The indication for this method thus also extends to organs that, because of a disorder, should not be palpated and mobilized directly. In this book, I introduce what I believe to be the most effective technique from the treatment concept according to Finet and Williame, namely expiratory dysfunction. I consider it particularly successful because the mobilizing effect is herein achieved by the diaphragm in the context of respiration, meaning that the patient's body is thus carrying out the real "work" itself.

In the circulatory movements according to **William A. Kuchera, DO,** and **Michael L. Kuchera, DO,** the osteopath does not aim at contact with the affected organ, but rather analyzes which arteries, veins, vegetative nerves, and lymphatic vessels supply an organ and dispose of its waste, using special techniques to influence the circulation of the organ. In this technique, the mobilization of the organ is not of primary importance. This concept is thus an excellent complement to the mobilizing concepts of Barral and Finet/Williame. These manipulations are less invasive and far too little known in some countries. For didactic reasons, I have recorded the appropriate techniques for each organ, knowing full well that an exact separation of its circulation and therefore an isolated treatment of an individual organ is not possible. The techniques themselves are described all together in the general section of the book.

The fourth treatment concept is the reflex therapy according to **Frank Chapman, DO.** The Chapman points are a valuable diagnostic tool, can provide follow-up results after treatment with visceral manipulation, and take advantage of the vegetative nervous system to influence the internal organs. Reflex therapy should be found in every therapeutic tool kit. The Chapman points have become highly valued tools for me.

These treatment techniques are supplemented by concise information about the physiology and clinical pathology of the individual organs. This information is not intended to be exhaustive but rather as a quick reference source in one's daily work.

While reading this book, you will encounter the term "central tendon" again and again. This is not to be confused with the "core link." That term is used in the English literature to refer to the connection between the base of the skull and the sacrum or coccyx via the dura mater. The central tendon, by contrast, refers to a fascial string that also runs through the body from the base of the skull to the pelvic floor, but is located anterior to the spinal column in the superficial and deeper-lying fascial layers of the body and does not include the dura mater. This fascial continuum works together as a functional unit: if a dysfunction is present in the body that should be protected in a global chain of protection, the central tendon can collaborate in this effort. The ability to carry out a fascial contraction is therefore of great importance. The fascia contracts towards the location of the dysfunction, thereby contributing to the protection of this area. As the fascial organ coverings (peritoneum, pericardium, pleura) are integrated into this system, compensatory increases in tension are also found in this fascia. As circulation passes through the fascia, elevated fascial tension disturbs the circulation of the tissue behind it. In concrete terms, this means that pathologic tension in the central tendon disturbs the circulation in the organs and can be the trigger point for impaired organ function or result in a reduced ability of the organ to compensate for biological, physical, or chemical noxa. Restoring normal tension in the central tendon is hence of vital importance for undisturbed organ function.

Contents

I Foundations and Techniques

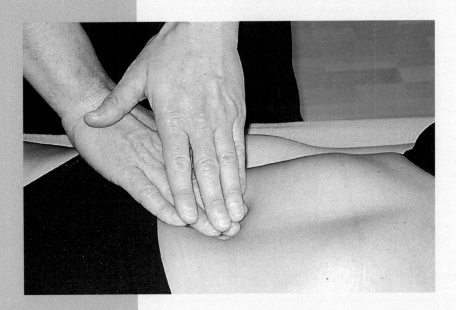

1 Visceral Manipulation according to Barral

Theory of Visceral Manipulation

■ Physiology of Organ Movement

We distinguish three movements of the internal organs: motricity, mobility, and motility.

Motricity

Motricity refers to passive changes in the position of the organs that result from arbitrary motor activity by the locomotor system.

If, for example, you bend the upper body to the right, the move compresses the abdominal organs on the right side but stretches the wall of the torso on the left, resulting in a pull on the left-sided organ attachments which enlarges their available space.

When bending the upper body forward, the intraperitoneal organs migrate anteriorly as the result of gravity and their high degree of mobility.

Any activity that involves continuous sitting compresses the small and large intestines and impairs their peristalsis.

Lifting both arms in maximum flexion results in an extension of the thoracic spinal column (TSC) and an inspiration position of the ribs. As the parietal pleura follows this movement of the thorax, and the lung is connected to the movement of the chest by its stretch, the lung increases its volume without having to make any additional respiratory effort.

Mobility

In visceral manipulation, mobility refers to the movement either between two organs or between an organ and the wall of the torso, the diaphragm, or another structure in the musculoskeletal system. The engine for this movement can be motricity or different "automatisms."

Automatism refers to a movement that is performed involuntarily by striated or smooth muscles. Furthermore we can differentiate between automatisms that occur continuously and movements of the organs marked by periodicity.

Automatisms include:
- diaphragmatic breathing
- heart action
- peristalsis of the visceral hollow organs in the gastrointestinal tract

Diaphragmatic breathing. With 12–14 breaths/min, the diaphragm contracts about 20 000 times a day. In doing so, it acts like a piston sliding up and down in a cylinder. During inspiration, the diaphragm sinks caudally, the volume of the thorax increases, and the abdominal organs migrate downward. The soft muscular abdominal wall allows the abdominal organs to move anteriorly out of the way; as a result, the volume of the abdomen hardly changes at all during inspiration.

During expiration, the opposite movement occurs.

Heart action. At 70 heartbeats/min, the heart contracts about 100 000 times a day. These actions act like vibrations on the mediastinal organs and, via the diaphragm, also on the abdomen.

Motility

Motility is defined as the intrinsic movement of the organs with a slow frequency and small amplitude. It can be detected by the hand of a trained practitioner and is the kinetic expression of movements in the organ tissues. During embryonic development, the evolving organs carry out growth movements and position shifts that remain stored in each organ cell as a kind of memory. Motility is a rhythmic repetition of this embryonic migration to its place of origin and back to the final, postnatal position.

Likewise, it is impossible to rule out a connection to the craniosacral rhythm, in spite of the fact that motility shows a different frequency.

We distinguish between a so-called expiration phase, that is, the movement toward the median line, and an inspiration phase, a movement in the opposite direction away from the median line.

The frequency is 7–8 cycles/min, one cycle comprising one expiration and one inspiration.

■ Visceral Joint

Motricity, automatisms, and mobility cause changes in positional relationships of the organs. The movement occurs along a defined axis with a defined amplitude and, thereby, the organs with structural relationships to each other act in a similar way to a joint in the locomotor system.

Two joint partners form the visceral joint; the two joint partners can be two organs (liver–kidney) or an organ and a muscular wall (liver–diaphragm).

The joint partners have surfaces that glide toward each other; the visceral joint partners are separated from each other by a capillary gap, and the surface of their gliding face is smooth and covered with a film of fluid.

The serous membranes—pleura, peritoneum, pericardium, and meninges/peripheral nerve sheaths—constitute most of these gliding surfaces.

The joint partners are fixed to each other: there are several attachments on the organs that are important for the axis of movement—see box.

Note

Organs are attached by:
- The double-leaf system
- The ligamentary system
- Turgor and intracavitary pressure
- The mesenteries
- The omenta

Double-Leaf System

Wherever we find a film of fluid (peritoneum, pleura, pericardium), the organs of a visceral joint are both separated from each other and connected by this fluid. They act in a similar way to two panes of glass with a drop of fluid between them—they can glide past each other, but the adhesive force keeps them together.

Ligamentary System

In visceral manipulation, ligaments are pleural or peritoneal folds that connect an organ to either the wall of the trunk or other organs. In most cases, they do not contain blood vessels but are sensitive and well innervated. They fix the organs against gravity.

Turgor and Intracavitary Pressure

Turgor or intravisceral pressure refers to the ability of an organ to occupy the largest space possible. The reasons for this characteristic are elasticity, vascular effects (decreased or increased blood circulation), and gases in hollow organs.

The intracavitary pressure is the sum of all intravisceral pressures plus the pressure between the organs.

This pressure causes the organs to be pressed and fixed against each other. As a result, we find a large excess of pressure in the abdomen, which is countered by a vacuum in the thorax. The diaphragm is the border layer between these pressure states. The organs near the diaphragm are influenced greatly by pressures. A diaphragmatic hernia will thus always lead to a movement of organ parts from the abdomen into the thorax, against

gravity. This illustrates the great potency of such pressure effects on the fixation of the organs.

Mesenteries

The mesenteries are duplicatures the peritoneum with only a minor role in fixation. They supply the organ's blood circulation.

Omenta

The omenta are also infoldings of the peritoneum that connect two organs to each other. Their role in organ fixation is rather small, although their vasculonervous function is of more importance.

■ Pathology of Organ Movement

Organs move around specific axes and with defined amplitudes. Changes in the axes of movement or amplitudes lead to deviations from the physiologic mobility or motility. Such changes lead to
- local pathologies first without and later with symptoms
- recurring local pathologies
- pathologies in visceral or parietal regions of the body that are linked via topographic, vascular, nervous, or fascial osteopathic chains

In principle, we distinguish between disturbed mobility and disturbed motility.

Disturbed Mobility

An organ completely or partly loses its ability to move as a result of the following causes.

Note

Causes of disturbed mobility:
- Adhesions/fixations
- Viscerospasm
- Ptosis

Articular restrictions. This dysfunction can lead to disturbed mobility and disturbed motility. If only the motility but not the mobility is disturbed, we speak of "adhesions." If, however, both movement qualities are impaired, we call this "fixations."

In fixations, the axis of movement and the amplitude could have changed. Causes include:
- infections
- inflammation
- surgical interventions
- blunt trauma

Muscular restrictions (viscerospasms). Viscerospasms affect only the hollow organs (e.g., stomach, intestines, or ureters). Irritation of the organ can lead to nonphysiologic contraction of the smooth muscles accompanied by impaired organ functions.

As a result, we notice a change in motility, especially in amplitude. Altered mobility affects the organ only when the viscerospasm has also adversely impacted the organ attachments.

Causes for irritations include:
- inflammation
- vegetative dysinnervation
- allergic reactions
- psychosomatic influences

Loss of ligamentary elasticity (ptosis). The loss of elasticity in ligamentary attachments causes diverse organs, such as the transverse colon, kidney, or urinary bladder, to descend with gravity.

The axes and amplitude of mobility change, as does motility, the causes of which include:
- a result of adhesions
- asthenic constitution
- anorexia or rapid weight loss due to other causes
- age-related loss of elasticity
- depression with generalized tonus reduction
- general laxity at the end of or after pregnancy
- delivery by vacuum extraction
- multiparity

Disturbed Motility

Motility can have its amplitude disturbed. The range of motion can be reduced in either one direction or both directions.

A disturbance also alters the rhythm of the movement:
- The rest phase between inspiration and expiration can be prolonged.
- We detect an arrhythmic motion.
- The frequency is reduced.

The causes include:
- general loss of vitality in the organ as a sign of pathology
- articular restriction
- ptosis
- viscerospasm

Diagnosis and General Treatment Principles in Visceral Osteopathy

■ Medical History

Questioning the patient allows the practitioner to collect information about the following keywords:
- current reason for consultation
- patient history with chronological list of items, for example:
  - accidents
  - operations
  - risk factors (pre-existing conditions, family history)
  - digestive and nutritional history
  - constipation
  - diarrhea
  - medication
- gynecologic history in women, for example:
  - irregular cycle
  - dysmenorrhea
  - birth control with intrauterine device (IUD) or the "pill"
- urologic history in men:
  - previous examinations
  - previous therapy

> **Note**
> - The patient history serves to put the practitioner on the right track.
> - Contraindications for osteopathic treatment should already have been identified.

■ Inspection

During an osteopathic inspection with the patient in the standing position, the following should be noted:
- asymmetric folds (e.g., gluteal fold)
- curvatures of the spine in three planes
- scars
- abdominal wall scoliosis
- upper abdomen protruding in the epigastric angle
- lower abdomen protruding
- trophic skin condition (e.g., color, circulation, rash)
- malpositions in the extremities
- abnormal posture, e.g.:
  - fallen arches, splay-foot, flat-foot
  - genu valgum or varum
  - malposition of the hip
  - pelvic asymmetries
  - malpositions in the ribs
  - funnel chest
  - pigeon chest
  - winged scapula
  - elevated shoulder
  - torticollis

- hyperlordosis
- hyperkyphosis
- malpositions of the head
- barrel-shaped thorax

Even this long list is not exhaustive. Ultimately, we look for findings that guide the practitioner to the dysfunctional organ or into the diagnostic zone.

In visceral manipulation, for example, we interpret posture abnormalities in light of the fact that the body creates convexities to compensate by allowing organs more room and concavities to compensate by providing protection to underlying structures.

Example of a Convexity

An upper abdomen that protrudes into the epigastric angle indicates dysfunction in the upper abdominal organs, which need space and move away anteriorly. When palpating this region, we are almost certain to find pain in individual organs, such as the stomach, or to trigger symptoms such as nausea.

Example of a Concavity

A left convex scoliosis with the vertex point of the concave curvature in the area of the right lower costal arch can indicate dysfunction in the liver or gallbladder. Compression of the organ by the concavity reduces mobility and provides rest or immobilization. This mechanism is comparable to a parietal joint that stops hurting when the person no longer moves it.

◼ Palpation

In palpation of the thorax, elasticity tests are performed at different locations on the ribs and sternum, to gain an impression of the fascial tensions in the ribcage.

Abdominal palpation is accomplished in two steps.

Superficial Palpation

During superficial palpation of the abdomen, the various regions of the abdomen (epigastrium, hypochondrium, etc.) are palpated with both hands in the fascial plane. This noteworthy layer consists of the fascia of the abdominal muscles, the greater omentum, and the parietal anterior peritoneum. To reach it in palpation, sink both hands into the abdomen until you detect the organs under your fingers. Then take the pressure off the abdomen just to the point where you no longer detect the organs.

Evaluate the patient for differences in tension between the two sides, triggering of pain by the palpation, and possibly evaluate existing scars for tension and sensitivity.

Deep Palpation

Deep palpation is applied to the organs themselves. We evaluate for:
- painfulness
- differences in tension
- position of the organ
- tone of the organ

Be particularly mindful of whether the palpation could cause parietal symptoms such as lumbalgia. This would indicate a possible causal link to the palpated organ.

In addition, pay attention to vegetative symptoms that can be triggered by the examination:
- nausea and vomiting
- sweating
- tachycardia
- tendency to collapse
- dizziness
- severe pain leading to tension that actively resists the palpation

These symptoms can be signs of acute disorders (e.g., cholecystitis) which are a contraindication to osteopathic treatment.

Caution!
If palpation or visceral manipulation triggers strong vegetative reactions, you must stop treatment and, if necessary, advise the patient to seek medical clarification.

◼ Inspection and Palpation Results

Inspection of the patient allows us to draw quite reliable conclusions about disturbed regions and dysfunctions of the body. In principle, you should focus on immediately noticeable abnormalities in posture, instead of searching for barely visible "minor details." The following is a discussion of some results of an inspection.

The position in which the patient holds the head allows us to draw important conclusions: ask the patient who is standing facing the examiner to close the eyes and bring the head to a position facing straight ahead. The patient may then open the eyes but should maintain the head position. If you now observe a clear tilt of the head with rotation and lateral inclination that deviate from the neutral position, this is a good indication of dysfunction in the head joints. It is not uncommon for this tilt to be combined with elevated shoulders, which in the author's eyes is merely a sign of hypertonicity in the trapezius muscle. The consequences of this head tilt can sometimes be far reaching for the abdomen: a blockage in the atlanto-occipital joint can lead to osseous narrowing of the jugular foramen directly, or we can see the build-up, e.g., in children, of constricting fascial trains on the jugular foramen as a result of malposition of the occiput. The jugular foramen is where the accessory, vagus, and glossopharyngeal nerves exit the base of the skull. The vagus and glossopharyngeal nerves have an important relationship with the internal organs—both have a role in the act of swallowing, and the vagus nerve is the parasympathetic nerve for the organs of the thorax and abdomen up to the Cannon–Böhm point. If these nerves are pinched in the jugular foramen, the viscera are also affected. We can cite baby colic, functional dyspepsia, and constipation as examples.

Malposition of the head can also be caused by the upper cervical spinal column (CSC). In particular, segments C2 and C3 are of interest for the internal organs. Articular blockage in these segments can lead to hypertonicity of the associated muscles at the segmental spinal cord level. This, in turn, affects the trapezius, which causes the apparent elevated shoulders.

It is therefore essential that the head joints and upper CSC be treated to create a parasympathetic compensation, which ultimately treats the organs.

The cervicothoracic transition is also an important area for the internal organs: it is common to find a hyperkyphosis at that position, which points to high fascial tension in the superior thoracic aperture. In the area of this hyperkyphosis, spider veins often appear as well, which should be understood as a sign of a circulatory problem in the superior thoracic aperture. In many patients, the greater supraclavicular fossa, an indentation posterior to the clavicle and anterior to the upper edge of the trapezius, is no longer an indentation but rather appears as a filled-in area, or even a "hill," and thus points to high fascial tension in the superior thoracic aperture.

In the thoracic aperture with the greater supraclavicular fossa, we find important circulatory structures for the thoracic and abdominal organs. On the left side, the thoracic duct drains into the venous angle formed by the internal jugular vein and the subclavian vein. The phrenic nerve runs along the anterior scalene muscle caudally and enters the thoracic aperture at the medial end of the clavicle. The vagus nerve takes a similar path into the thorax near the sternal end of the clavicle. If these structures are irritated by high fascial tension, this can affect the organs in the thorax or abdomen: it can, for example, impair lymphatic drainage from the abdomen, the function of the diaphragm, or the vagus supply area.

The brachial plexus and the subclavian vein traverse the thoracic aperture, run across the first rib and below the clavicle in the direction of the axilla, and continue into the arm. Deep inside the fossa, we find the stellate ganglion, which not only provides sympathetic fibers for the heart but also supplies the mucous membranes of the head and sympathetically the arm. Similar to the circulatory structures mentioned above, these vessels and nerves can also be pinched as a result of fascial hypertonicity in the thoracic aperture. Heart irritation, thoracic

outlet syndrome, and chronic sinusitis could be possible consequences.

Furthermore, diverse circulation-related syndromes of the arm have a cause in the viscera. Irritations of the sensitive fibers of the phrenic nerve, as, for example, caused by pericarditis, distension of the Glisson capsule, or cholecystitis, can tonify the segmental muscles via a viscerosomatic reflex. If the subclavius is affected, the brachial plexus or subclavian vein can be pinched because this muscle brings the clavicle and the first rib close to each other. The result can be different circulatory syndromes of the arm, such as Sudeck syndrome, Dupuytren contracture, or medial and lateral epicondylitis.

Irritation of the stellate ganglion can likewise lead to high fascial tension in the superior thoracic aperture, with functional problems in the area of the head, e.g., dry eyes or chronic sinusitis.

An increased cervical kyphosis often stems from a posture with flexed thorax and protracted shoulders. In physiotherapy, this is called sternosymphyseal strain position, which expresses the fact that the distance between the sternum and symphysis is shortened. In osteopathy, we interpret this as a sign of a shortened central tendon.

The central tendon is a fascial cord that runs from the skull base through the body down to the pelvic floor and collaborates as a functional unit in such a way that the fasciae contract toward the location with the greatest tension. Therefore locations with high fascial tension are fields of interference that the body is trying to normalize, or express an attempt to compensate by developing independent high fascial tension. In this respect, the central tendon tries to set up a mechanism, that is, a protective mechanism for dysfunctional body regions, but can itself build up high tension within its fascia.

The posture described above thus indicates that the central tendon has contracted because of a location with high tension. This location can be in the thorax, which we would recognize from the fact that there would be a mild funnel chest, or in the abdomen, in which case both the look of the back and the shape of the abdomen give clues as to the location of the tension.

For the osteopath, scoliotic malpositions also indicate places of high tension. As already suggested above, we speak of a diagnostic angle, which is found at the vertex of the spinal column curve. The concavity is viewed as the place with the highest fascial tension. At this concave side, the space for an organ is reduced to immobilize it in a type of protective mechanism. On the other hand, it is also possible that an organ has to occupy more space on the convex side, e.g., because it is swollen as the result of inflammation. An increased lordosis should be interpreted accordingly.

High internal abdominal tension can also be recognized from the shape of the abdomen. An abdomen that visibly protrudes below the costal arch in the upper abdomen (like a terrace or step) must be interpreted as a sign of dysfunction in one or several upper abdominal organs.

If the upper abdomen is flat but the abdomen protrudes from the navel down to the symphysis like a ball, this could be caused by ptosis of the small intestine. This is accompanied by increased lordosis in the upper lumbar spinal column (LSC). The small intestine is suspended via the root of the mesentery. The root is attached indirectly in the cranial part through L2 and L3. If the small intestine gradually starts drooping, the LSC forms a lordosis as compensation. To gain more certainty here, place the fingertips on the spinous processes of the upper LSC and lift the abdomen slightly anteriorly above the symphysis, without causing the patient to lose balance. If you feel that the vertebrae of the LSC push slightly against your fingers, i.e., flex, this confirms your visual finding.

You will notice again and again that there are two types of abdomens. There are solid bulging abdomens that look like a ball. When you palpate such abdomens, the pressure inside the abdomen is so high that you can barely put your hand into the belly. Such abdomens are found almost exclusively in men. It may be tempting to say that these men are simply overweight, but you will notice further that they commonly do not suffer from major fat accumulation in the subcutaneous tissue, so we cannot speak of overweight in general. Excess fat is stored primarily on the inside of the abdomen: the greater omentum, liver, or appendages of the colon (epiploic appendices) are the preferred locations. Apparently, this special "male" type of fat deposit is related to the hormone testosterone.

Nevertheless, the shape of the abdomen has far-reaching functional effects: the diaphragm, for example, is forced to perform its respiratory function against clearly increased pressure in the abdomen. As a result, the accessory respiratory muscles are forced to work harder. The scalene muscle consequently becomes hypertonic and triggers compression syndromes in the brachial plexus and the subclavian artery, the so-called thoracic outlet syndrome. The high pressure in the abdomen also has an effect posteriorly. Thus, this pressure can fix herniated disks in such a way that the nucleus pulposus is no longer able to glide back anteriorly.

A different shape abdomen is more frequently found in women. The abdomen as a whole is soft and easy to palpate for diagnosis and treatment, even though it can also be a large belly. The fat is not, however, deposited on the inside of the abdomen but rather in the subcutaneous tissue. This difference is explained by hormonal reasons. In general, female sex hormones are a predisposing factor for several female visceral problems: women are much more likely to have ptoses of the organs than men.

Spider veins can form in the area of the costal arch, as in the thoracocervical transition. These veins run unilaterally or bilaterally below the nipple in a lateral-to-caudal arch. They almost trace the attachment of the diaphragm and are thus an expression of a diaphragmatic dysfunction.

We can see comparable vein patterns on the sacrum and in the lumbosacral transition as a sign of circulatory congestion in the small pelvis. Sometimes you have to ask the patient to bend forward to make these lumbosacral spider veins appear more clearly. Additional clues for stopped circulation in the pelvic area are a tendency to leg edema, marbled skin, or skin color in the legs that does not match the rest of the body. In this case, the legs are colored pale blue compared with the upper body. If you look at the patient from behind, the impression is that the upper body does not match the lower body. The upper body is slender, so you would expect a small pelvis and slim legs, but the pelvis is broad and the legs very stocky. In this visual finding, congestion will have developed in the pelvis over a long period of time and changed the lower body. When you ask the patient whether their figure has always looked like this, they often say no and cite pregnancy, for example, as the moment of change.

■ Listening Tests according to Barral

Listening Test in Standing Position

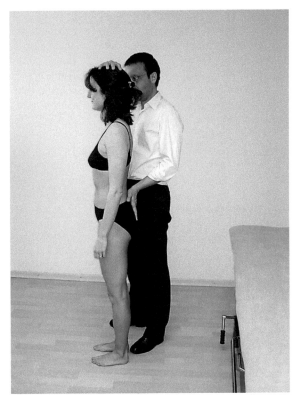

Fig. 1.1

Starting Position
The patient stands with the legs hip-width apart, the arms hanging loosely by the sides of the body, and the eyes closed. The practitioner stands to the side of the patient and places one hand with no pressure on the head, and the other hand, also with no pressure, on the sacrum. The practitioner's hands serve only to stabilize the patient.

Procedure
Ask the patient to "let themself hang," not to fix one posture by muscle strength but to follow any tensions and allow the body to sink into a fascially "decompressed" (in the literal sense of the word) position. Be mindful not to help the patient into a certain position.

Evaluation
The area of greatest concavity is the diagnostic zone in which we can assume that a dysfunction is present.

Listening Test in Seated Position

Starting Position
The patient is seated; the legs do not touch the floor. The practitioner stands to the side of the patient.

Procedure
Corresponds to the procedure in the standing position.

Evaluation
For the test in the seated position, the lower extremity is "switched off," i.e., the test provides information from the pelvis up cranially.

Listening Test in Supine Position

"Leg Pull"

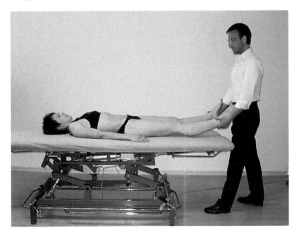

Fig. 1.2

Starting Position
The patient is in supine position, legs stretched out. The practitioner stands at the foot of the table.

Procedure
Take both of the patient's heels and lift the legs slightly up off the table. In turn, pull each leg in its perpendicular axis caudally, evaluate the fascial tensions, and observe how the pull progresses cranially.

Evaluation
The side with the higher tension is the dysfunctional side. If the pull does not proceed harmonically from the leg through the pelvis cranially, you can look for the diagnostic zone in the place where the pull motion stops.

"Arm Pull"

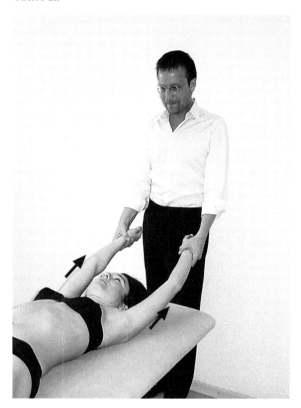

Fig. 1.3

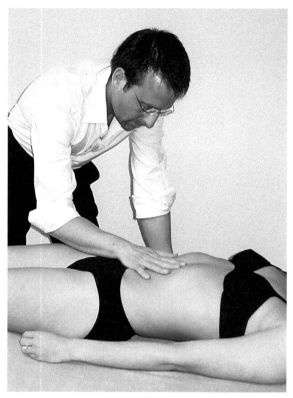

Fig. 1.4

Starting Position
The patient is in supine position, legs stretched out. The practitioner stands at the head of the table.

Procedure
Take both the patient's hands and pull the arms in their perpendicular axes cranially, evaluate the fascial tensions, and observe how the pull progresses caudally.

Evaluation
The side with the higher tension is the dysfunctional side. If the pull does not proceed harmonically from the arm through the thorax caudally, look for the diagnostic zone in the place where the pull motion stops.

Starting Position
The patient is in the supine position, legs stretched out. The practitioner stands next to the patient.

Procedure
Place one hand flat on the patient's abdomen, with the palm lying on the navel. Apply enough pressure for the palpation to reach the superficial fascial plane.

Evaluation
You will notice the movement of the fascia. Follow this movement to find the diagnostic zone.

> **Note**
> Great tension develops at the location where a dysfunction is present. The fascia moves toward the place of greatest tension, which is also the diagnostic zone.

Sotto–Hall Test according to Barral

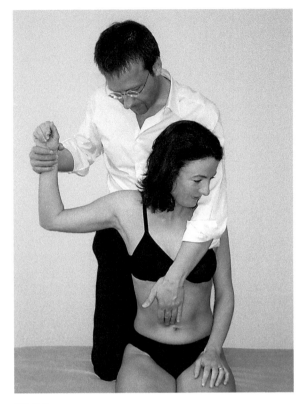

Fig. 1.5

Starting Position
The patient is seated on the table; the legs do not touch the floor. The practitioner stands behind the patient.

Procedure
Take one of the patient's hands and palpate the radial pulse. Then guide the arm into 90° abduction and maximal outward rotation. As the last step, bring the patient's head into contralateral rotation. This means that if the right arm is brought into position, the head is turned to the left and rotated.

Evaluation
If the pulse disappears in this position, the test is positive. The fascia in the greater supraclavicular fossa is brought under so much tension that the subclavian artery is compressed until the pulse is no longer palpable.

Reasons for this high fascial tension can be parietal, e.g., thoracic spinal column (TSC) dysfunctions, but also visceral—the osteopathic dysfunction of an organ, e.g., fixation, is conducted via a fascial chain up into the superior thoracic aperture and causes the positive test result.

To differentiate the affected organ, complete this test. Maintain the arm and head position while applying mild pressure to the organs in which you suspect that you will find the disturbance; perform an inhibition. If the pulse now returns, you have identified the dysfunctional organ. The inhibition in effect removes the organ from the fascial chain, as a result of which fascial tension drops and the subclavian artery is no longer compressed.

In general, we can say that the right arm serves as the test arm for the right side of the trunk, and the left arm for the left side. Nevertheless, do not take this division too seriously because there are also abdominal organs that are not paired.

This test is also referred to as the completed Adson–Wright test.

Rebound Test according to Barral

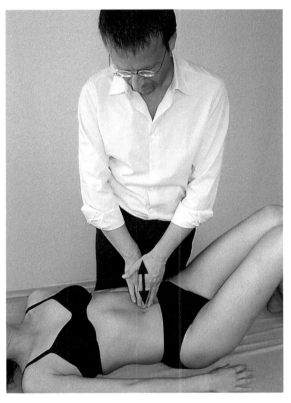

Fig. 1.6

Starting Position
The patient is in the supine position, legs bent. The practitioner stands next to the patient.

Procedure
With hands on top of each other, the practitioner presses into the patient's abdomen on an organ and abruptly lets go.

Evaluation
If pressure on the organ is painful, the disturbance is located in the organ itself, e.g., as an inflammation or spasm.

If, however, release of the pressure is painful, the cause is to be found in the attachments of the organ.

This test can also be performed in other starting positions, e.g., in a seated position.

Example. Lift the liver up against the diaphragm; compress it. The occurrence of any pain leads to the conclusion that the cause is in the organ itself.

Subsequently, release the pressure and let the liver fall back caudally. If the pain occurs at this point, the attachments of the liver are irritated, e.g., ligament fibrosis.

■ Completed Tests according to Barral

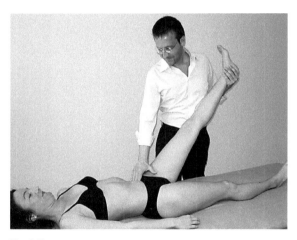

Fig. 1.7

The principle of the completed test consists of a control finding related to the reason for the consultation, e.g., painful rotational limitations of the TSC, and achieving improvement in this finding by means of organ inhibition.

Such control findings can be:
- impaired mobility in parietal joints with or without pain
- fascial tension in the extremities or trunk
- sensitivity to pressure in the ligaments, bursae, tendons, or other soft-tissue structures

Example. The reason for the consultation is lumboischialgia with radiating pain in the right posterior thigh. The fascial tension in the right leg is the control finding.

Hold the right extended leg by the foot and lift it off the table until you can feel fascial resistance against the lift. Hold the leg steady in this position and, using pressure, inhibit an organ related to the lumboischialgia, e.g., the ascending colon.

If the fascial tension is reduced during the inhibition, you can guide the leg further into the flexion until it reaches the new fascial barrier. Just as in the Sotto–Hall test,

the inhibition removes the organ from the fascial chain, as a result of which fascial tension drops in the leg.

The inhibited organ was contributing to the lumboischialgia.

■ Ventilation Test according to Barral

If a deep inspiration causes pain in the abdomen, the organ itself can be the reason for the consultation.

If, however, it is the deep expiration that is painful, suspect a problem with the attachments of one or several organs.

■ Hyperextension Test according to Barral

The practitioner helps the sitting patient into maximum extension of the spinal column. This movement exerts a pull on the attachments of the abdominal organs. If these attachments are fibrosed or sticky, this could trigger pain in the abdominal region.

■ General Treatment Principles and Possibilities in Visceral Treatment

In visceral manipulation, the five principles of osteopathy form the foundation of any work:
1. The holistic view of the human body—the principle of holism.
2. Life is movement.
3. Autoregulation of the body.
4. Structure and function depend on each other.
5. Circulation—the body's juices must flow.

The practitioner draws conclusions about the dysfunctions of the body based on the osteopathic diagnosis and its analysis. When an organ has been identified as the cause of the complaint, the practitioner attempts to restore the physiologic three-dimensional mobility of the organ through visceral manipulation.

In this process, all aspects of organ dynamics come into play:
- mobility
- motility
- fascial movement

Likewise, circulation in its broadest sense should be improved, improving the organ's trophic state:
- blood circulation
- lymph flow
- neurovegetative impulse

The practitioner treats the organ *in situ* and hopes that it will result in improved function, e.g., you can mobilize the large intestine to treat chronic constipation. This process of improving function requires time, which the body uses to apply its self-healing powers.

The success of osteopathic treatment in women with menstruation-related lower back pain can, for example, be evaluated only after a menstrual cycle has completed. As a result, between 2 and 4 weeks can pass between two visceral treatment sessions.

> **Note**
> The five principles of osteopathy:
> 1. The holistic view of the human body—the principle of holism.
> 2. Life is movement.
> 3. Autoregulation of the body.
> 4. Structure and function depend on each other.
> 5. Circulation—the body's juices must flow.

■ Possibilities in Visceral Manipulation

Reflex Point Treatment according to Barral

Reflex points are those anatomic structures in the gastrointestinal tract that function as sphincters. These reflex points include the following:
- gastroesophageal transition
- cardia
- pylorus
- major duodenal papilla
- duodenojejunal flexure
- ileocecal valve
- pelvic floor

These anatomic structures are often clearly sensitive to pressure. When treating a reflex point, this causes noticeable relaxation and reduction of pain in the sphincter itself and also in other areas of the gastrointestinal tract. It is most likely the viscerovisceral reflexes and special anatomic characteristics in these reflex points that are responsible for this reaction.

Principles

In this book, we discuss treatments for the reflex points 3–6. They follow the same principles:
- Palpate into the depth of the abdomen at the place where the reflex point projects onto the abdominal wall until you feel the reflex point.
- You can now treat the sphincter with friction in a clockwise direction, vibrations, inhibitions, or rebound (see below).
- Continue treating until relaxation occurs or the sensitivity of the point is noticeably reduced.
- Reflex point treatment can be done at the start of a visceral manipulation to achieve general relaxation of the viscera.

Inhibitions

Inhibitions are constant applications of pressure on a structure. Reflexogenically, they cause detonification and pain reduction at the treated point.

The inhibition is sustained for between 30 seconds and 2 minutes.

Rebound Technique

In this treatment method, you compress parts of an organ or stretch its attachments to the maximum extent possible. Then you abruptly release the structure and repeat the whole procedure several times.

This is a good method for detonifying a spasm or mobilizing adhesions or fixations.

Treatment of Mobility

Mobility is improved by manually supporting an organ directly or indirectly in its physiologic movement in three dimensions.

If you find, for example, impairment of liver mobility in the frontal plane, treat this movement in its full range of movement in accordance with principles similar to those for mobilizing a parietal joint—one joint partner is the fixed point, the other the mobile point. These two points can also be interchanged, or both partners can become mobile points. Pay attention to the axes and planes of movement that need improvement.

Direct Treatment

Place your hands on the organ and directly mobilize the structure.

Indirect Treatment

Mobilize the organ by means of levers, e.g., you can use the ribs as levers to mobilize the liver three-dimensionally (see below).

Direct and indirect techniques can be combined.

Treatment of Motility according to Barral

Principle

Starting Position
Place your hand without pressure on the patient's abdomen in the area of the organ that requires treatment. The forearm rests on the abdomen. Assume a relaxed sitting position.

Test Procedure

When you can feel the motility movement, evaluate the amplitude and direction of the inspiration and expiration movements, as well as the rhythm of the movement as a whole. If a disturbance is present in one or both aspects of the motility movement, treat the patient.

Treatment

Motility is treated indirectly by following the unimpaired movement, remaining at the end-point of this movement for several cycles, and then following the impaired movement to the new end-point.

You can also try to increase the free movement in its range (induction). Subsequently, check whether the impaired movement direction has improved.

Repeat this movement again and again until the motility has returned to normal in terms of rhythm, direction, and amplitude.

2 Fascial Treatment of the Organs according to Finet and Williame

Foundations

The body's fascia consists of connective tissue and forms a continuum. In this context, we can distinguish superficial, middle, and deep fascia, but all layers are connected to each other and form a unit in the craniocaudal and anteroposterior directions.

We can thus draw the following conclusion: a disturbance of the fascial dynamic anywhere in the body will, over time, cause a response in all fascia. This means that a dysfunction in a deep-lying area of the body's fascia can be detected in superficial tissue.

> **Note**
> - The body's fascia connects different tissues to each other.
> - It responds to disturbing factors as a unit.
> - A pathologic fascial pull in the depth of the body can also be detected as a disturbance in the superficial fascia.

The fascial dynamic can be disturbed by the following:
- adhesions (as a result of surgery, inflammation, or blunt trauma)
- ptoses
- viscerospasms
- parietal dysfunctions
- craniosacral dysfunctions

Disturbance of the fascial dynamic has consequences for the neurovegetative and hemodynamic supply of the organ:
- The circulatory conduits penetrate the organ's fascia to reach the organ.
- An additional vicious cycle results: if a disturbance of the fascia negatively affects the trophic state of an organ, the organ functions will be impaired, and the fascia responds in turn with an aphysiologic pull.
- Aphysiologic tissue pulls in the fascia also impair the mobility and motility of an organ. This can lead to functional impairments in the organ or parietal symptoms.

We can cite adhesions in the area of the small intestine after abdominal surgery as an example: the intestinal loops attach to the abdominal wall or to each other, and we see digestive problems or lumbar pain.

> **Note**
> An impaired fascial dynamic has neurovegetative and hemodynamic consequences for organs. The mobility and motility can also change.

Principles of Diagnosis

The superficial fascia reacts to dysfunctions in the lower layers of the fascia with a change in tissue pull.

It is the goal of visceral diagnosis of the fascia to obtain information about the lower-lying organ fascia by palpating the superficial fascial tissue pulls (induction test) and by neurovegetative reactions (hemodynamic test).

By testing the superficial fascia in the abdominal wall, we identify the disturbed organ.

Principles of Fascial Organ Treatment

The diaphragm is the engine of fascial movement in the abdominal organs. Migration of the organs caudally during inhalation also includes a fascial movement caudally in the abdomen. In addition to this caudal movement, the individual organ fascia carries out concomitant rotations.

For the purpose of treatment, we use the respiratory movement as the mobilizing element.

Normalization aims at restoring the physiologic fascial dynamic of the organ by mobilizing the superficial abdominal fascia. In this way, each organ has its specific direction for mobilization, which is discussed further in the chapters about individual organs in Section 2.

Principles of the Technique for Expiratory Dysfunction

Any fascial techniques of Finet and Williame that we discuss in this book consist of treatment for expiratory dysfunctions.

Place your hands in the diagnostic zone of the organ and apply pressure posteriorly until you palpate the superficial fascial plane.

You have reached the correct treatment plane when at a depth just before feeling the organs. To make it easier, first palpate more deeply into the abdomen until you feel the organs and then back off a little.

During inhalation, both hands simultaneously pull caudally and, if appropriate, into the organ-specific rotation. During expiration, you maintain the position that you have reached. Repeat this procedure until you reach the end of the fascial movement. The pull is then released during the next expiration.

Repeat this procedure four or five times.

Contraindications

- acute abdomen
- carcinoma
- gallstones
- aortic aneurysm

Hemodynamic Test

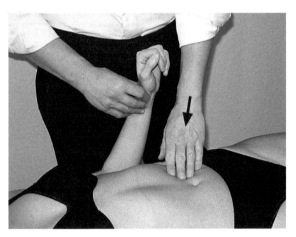

Fig. 2.1

Starting Position
The patient is in the supine position, legs stretched out. The practitioner stands next to the patient.

Procedure
With one hand, feel the patient's radial pulse. Place the other hand in the diagnostic zone of the organ in question and apply mild pressure posteriorly.

Testing Sequence
If the pulse drops temporarily during this pressure on the abdomen, this is the normal response—the test is negative and the organ not disturbed. Sometimes it also happens that the pulse fails to drop when you apply pressure to the abdomen but temporarily accelerates as you release the pressure. In either case, we can interpret this as a physiologic reaction to the pulse.

If, however, the pulse fails to respond with a change when we either apply or release the pressure, the test is positive—the organ's fascia is disturbed.

During this test, it is important that the applied pressure is not too strong.

This test is explained by neurovegetative reflexes via baroreceptors.

Fascial Induction Test

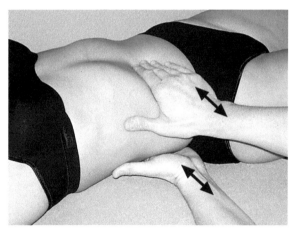

Fig. 2.2

Starting Position
The patient is in the supine position, legs stretched out. The practitioner stands next to the patient.

Procedure
Place both hands as follows on the abdomen.

Transverse Shift
One hand lies anterior on the diagnostic zone of the organ, the other posterior at the same level.

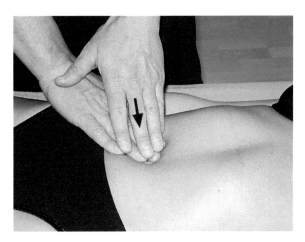

Fig. 2.3

Anterior–Posterior Induction
Both hands lie on top of each other on the organ's diagnostic zone.

Testing Sequence
During the transverse shift, both hands carry out a transverse displacement of the superficial fascia; during the anterior–posterior induction, they apply light pressure in the plane of the superficial fascia.

The object of the evaluation is the tension of the fascia and its dynamics; a free and harmonic motion in a consistent state of tension is normal.

In a second step, abruptly release the pressure without completely moving the hands out of the palpation. Evaluate the rebound of the fascia laterally or anteriorly: if the organ is not disturbed, the fascia should rebound like a tightly stretched trampoline.

If you detect higher tensions in the path of the movement, a disharmonic motion (clipped, halting, restricted), or just dogged rebound of the fascia (like an insufficiently stretched trampoline) during this test, the organ is disturbed.

3 Circulatory Techniques according to Kuchera

Objective

An organ can be influenced by its circulation, which includes the arterial, venous, and lymphatic systems, as well as the sympathetic and parasympathetic innervations.

By means of the following treatment techniques, we can affect the trophic state of the organ. This is very important for organs that show pathology, e.g., gastritis.

A prerequisite for these techniques is familiarity with circulatory anatomy, which is discussed in the chapters on individual organs.

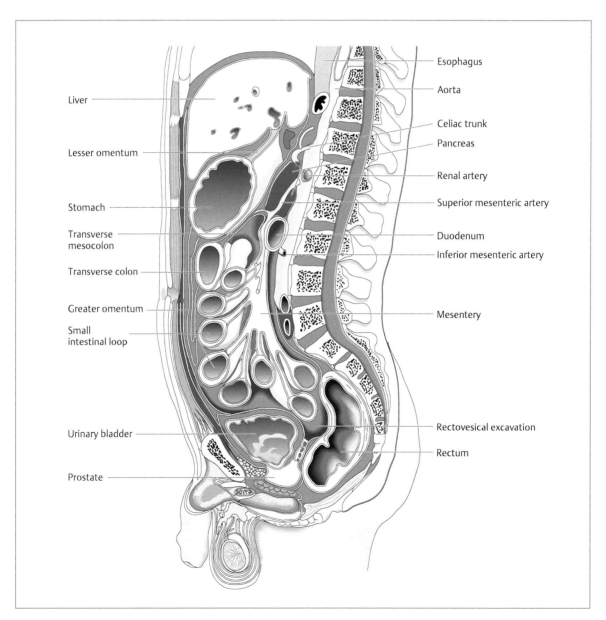

Fig. 3.1 The abdomen in sagittal section.

Principle of the Techniques

Arterial Stimulation

The large vessel trunks for the abdominal space lie in front of the abdominal aorta and hence in front of the spinal column. Treating the spinal column (manipulation, mobilization, etc.) at the corresponding height stimulates the arterial supply of attached organs.

> **Note**
> The celiac trunk supplies the upper abdominal organs— the liver, gallbladder, stomach, spleen, and pancreas— and the start of the duodenum. It is located approximately at the level of T12–L1.

> **Note**
> The superior mesenteric artery supplies the duodenum, jejunum, ileum, cecum, and colon up to the Cannon– Böhm point on the transverse colon. It lies approximately at the level of L1–L2.

> **Note**
> The inferior mesenteric artery supplies the colon from the Cannon–Böhm point on up to the upper section of the rectum. It lies at the level of L3–L4.

Venous Stimulation

The organs of the gastrointestinal tract drain their blood into the portal vein before it flows out through the liver into the inferior vena cava. Techniques that positively affect the portal vein, liver, or diaphragm improve venous drainage from the gastrointestinal tract.

Lymphatic Stimulation

All techniques that promote lymphatic drainage improve the trophic state of the organ, e.g., diaphragm techniques, grand maneuver, etc.

Vegetative Harmonization

Parasympathetic. Techniques that treat the vagus or sacral parasympathetic nerve have a harmonizing effect on the internal organs, e.g., craniosacral techniques, treatment of the larynx, mediastinum techniques, etc.

Sympathetic. On the basis of familiarity with the innervation of the organ, treatments that harmonize at the sympathetic level follow the course of the sympathetic nerves or plexus, e.g., sympathetic trunk stimulation by means of the rib-raise technique, diaphragm techniques, or stimulation of the prevertebral ganglia.

Techniques

Vegetative Harmonization

Rib-Raise Technique

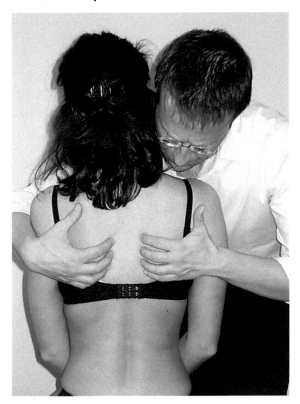

Fig. 3.2

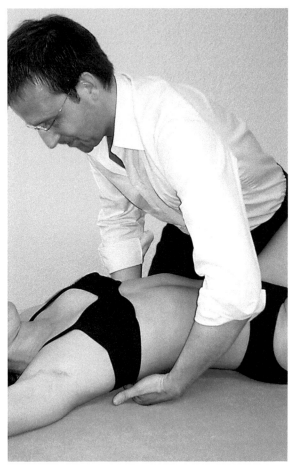

Fig. 3.3

Starting Position

The patient is in the supine position, legs stretched out, arms at the sides of the body. The practitioner stands to the side of the patient.

Procedure

Using the fingertips of both hands, make contact with the skin area lateral to the transverse process above the ribs.

Place the fingers on both sides in such a way that the patient's thorax is lifted passively off the table.

Treatment

Maintain this position until fascial release takes place. Then shake the patient's thorax rhythmically above the positioned fingers 8–10 times for sympathetic stimulation.

> **Note**
> The sympathetic trunk with its ganglia is located in front of the heads of the ribs.

Treatment of the Preaortic Plexus

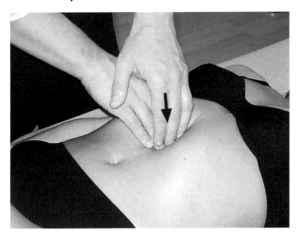

Fig. 3.4

Treatment of the Ischiorectal Fossa

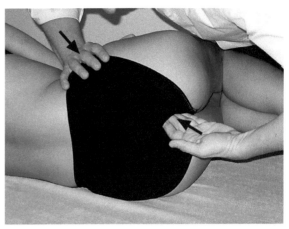

Fig. 3.6

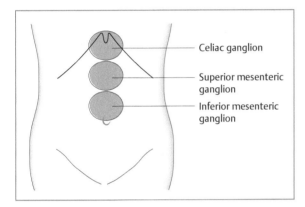

Celiac ganglion

Superior mesenteric ganglion

Inferior mesenteric ganglion

Fig. 3.5 Projection of the prevertebral plexus onto the abdominal wall.

Starting Position

The patient is in the supine position. The practitioner stands next to the patient.

Procedure

At the height of the projection of the preaortic plexus on the abdominal wall, place the fingers of both hands next to each other in the center line and let them sink into the depth of the abdomen until you reach the plexus. It may be necessary to stop repeatedly on the way in and await fascial release.

Treatment

When you have arrived at the plexus, maintain pressure until you have obtained fascial release. Then stimulate the preaortic plexus by means of repeated rebounds.

Starting Position

The patient is in the lateral position, hip and knees bent to 90°; the side to be treated faces up. The practitioner stands behind the patient.

Procedure

Place the fingers of the caudal hand medial to the ischiadic tuber and lateral to the coccyx, near the tuber, with the palm facing up. The cranial hand grips the iliac crest from anterior near the anterosuperior iliac spine (ASIS).

Treatment

The caudal hand exerts careful pressure cranially and anteriorly (in the approximate direction of the cranial hand). Wait for fascial release and then increase the pressure. The pressure of the caudal hand is applied in the direction of the greatest fascial tension. The cranial hand maintains counterpressure. You can work with careful vibrations.

> **Note**
> In the ischiorectal/ischioanal fossa, you find the pudendal canal (the Alcock canal) with the internal pudendal veins, pudendal nerve, and posterior nerves of the penis/clitoris.

Larynx Mobilization

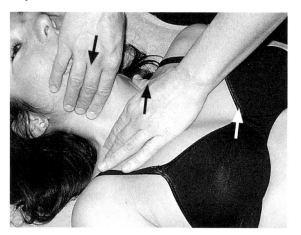

Fig. 3.7

Starting Position

The patient is in the supine position. The practitioner stands by the side of the patient.

Procedure

The practitioner's cranial hand fixates the mandible with the thumb and two or three fingers. The caudal hand lies with the thumb and two or three fingers on the floor of the mouth.

Treatment

The caudal hand mobilizes the floor of the mouth with translatoric pushes; the cranial hand fixates. As muscles and fascia relax, both hands move on caudally, proceeding in the same manner. The cranial hand can also alternate with the caudal hand in the mobilization.

When both hands lie on the neck, they must grip gently but also deeply enough to mobilize the larynx and the deep neck fascia. This has a positive effect on the deep vessel–nerve path with the vagus nerve.

Mediastinum Mobilization according to Barral

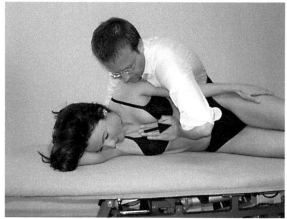

Fig. 3.8

Starting Position

The patient is in the lateral position. The practitioner stands behind the patient.

Procedure

The practitioner places the anterior hand on the lower third of the patient's sternum, with the fingertips pointing cranially. The posterior hand, also with the fingertips pointing cranially, lies on the spinal column at the level of the sternal manubrium.

Treatment

With the anterior hand, apply pressure caudally and posteriorly; with the posterior hand, apply pressure cranially and anteriorly. Both hands release pressure simultaneously and abruptly (rebound). Repeat this process 8–10 times. Then position the hands in such a way that the anterior hand lies on the manubrium and the posterior hand on the spinal column at the level of the lower third of the sternum. Now apply pressure with the anterior hand in a cranial–posterior direction and with the posterior hand in a caudal–anterior direction.

> **Note**
> Many structures with circulatory significance for the thoracic and abdominal organs are located in the mediastinum:
> - Sympathetic trunk
> - Vagus nerve
> - Aorta
> - Thoracic duct

Oscillations on the Sacrum

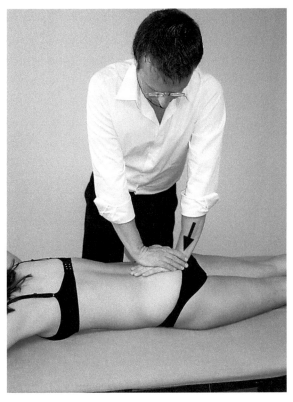

Fig. 3.9

Starting Position
The patient is in the prone position. The practitioner stands next to the patient.

Procedure
Place both hands on top of each other on the lower third of the sacrum and apply pressure cranially and anteriorly.

Treatment
Release and exert rhythmic pressure: oscillate on the sacrum with a frequency of 150–180/min. Apply this impulse for about 2 min.

> **Note**
> Vegetative ganglia, plexus, and nerves are located anterior to the sacrum, together with arteries and veins for the pelvic organs.

Intraosseous Technique on the Sacrum

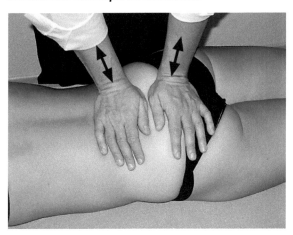

Fig. 3.10

Starting Position
The patient lies in the prone position. The practitioner stands next to the patient.

Procedure
Place both hands on the sacrum, with the thenar eminences next to each other. The transition zone between two segments of the sacrum lies in between.

Treatment
Apply intermittent pressure with the hands to the sacrum and create an intraosseous arc tension. Length of treatment: 1–2 min.

Lymphatic Stimulation

Sternal Pump and Recoil on the Sternum

Oscillations on the Sternum

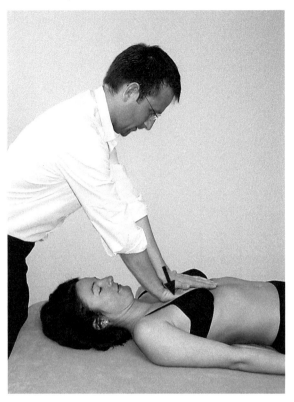

Fig. 3.11

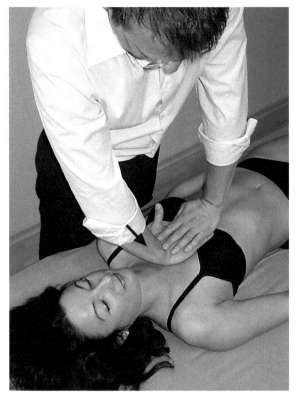

Fig. 3.12

Starting Position
The patient is in the supine position. The practitioner stands at the head of the table.

Procedure
Place both hands on top of each other on the sternum, with the thenar eminence on the sternal angle.

Treatment
Ask the patient to inhale deeply. During the deep exhalation, apply pressure with both hands caudally and posteriorly. Release the pressure on the next inhalation. Repeat this process five to six times.
　You can conclude this pump technique with a recoil.

Starting Position
The patient is in the supine position. The practitioner stands to the side of the patient.

Procedure
Place both hands on top of each other on the sternum, with the thenar eminence on the sternal angle.

Treatment
Both hands apply rhythmic pressure to the sternum in a caudal–posterior direction. The frequency is 150–180/min for a duration of about 2 min.

Abdominal Vibrations

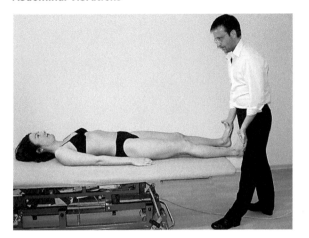

Fig. 3.13

Grand Maneuver

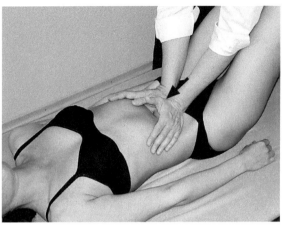

Fig. 3.14

Starting Position
The patient is in the supine position. The practitioner stands at the foot of the table.

Procedure
Take hold of the patient's feet from plantar at the toes and metatarsal heads, and push them in posterior extension to the limit of the motion.

Treatment
Now apply rhythmic impulses in the direction of the posterior extension with a frequency of 150–180/min for about 2 min. The vibrations should be strong enough that you can easily see them at the patient's head.

Starting Position
The patient is in the supine position. The practitioner stands to the side of the patient.

Procedure
With both hands, reach into the abdomen medial to the iliac wings, to hold the entire intestinal system between your hands.

Treatment
Ask the patient to inhale deeply. During exhalation, push the intestines cranially underneath the diaphragm. Release pressure on the next inhalation. Repeat this five to six times.

Then stop, releasing the pressure during the inhalation phase and again increase the pressure during the exhalation. Repeat this increase cycle two or three times. Finally, at the start of an inhalation phase, abruptly release the pressure.

Oscillations on Top of the Liver	*Stretching the Hepatoduodenal Ligament*

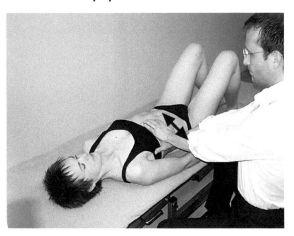

Fig. 3.15

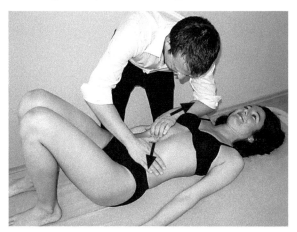

Fig. 3.16

Starting Position
The patient is in the supine position. The practitioner stands on the patient's right side.

Procedure
Place both hands laterally on the right half of the thorax in the area of the liver.

Treatment
Now apply rhythmic impulses medially with a frequency of 150–180/min for about 2 min.

Starting Position
The patient is in the supine position. The practitioner stands on the patient's right side.

Procedure
With the cranial hand, grasp the skin below the right costal arch. Set your lower arm down on the thorax in such a way that the elbow is pointing to the patient's right shoulder. The caudal hand touches the abdomen about five finger-widths (patient's fingers) cranial from the navel and about two finger-widths to the right of the center line. Let the caudal hand sink slowly into the depth of the abdomen.

Treatment
Pull both hands diagonally away from each other—the cranial hand toward the right shoulder and the caudal hand toward the patient's navel.

> **Note**
> Three important circulatory structures run in the hepatoduodenal ligament:
> 1. Portal vein.
> 2. Proper hepatic artery.
> 3. Common bile duct.

Diaphragm Technique

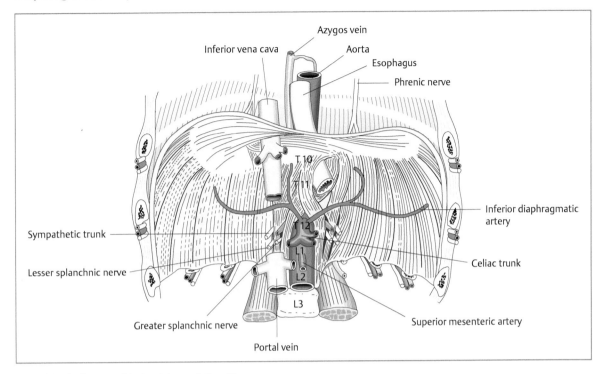

Fig. 3.17 Diaphragm with circulatory relationships.

Mobilization of the Lower Ribs in Translation

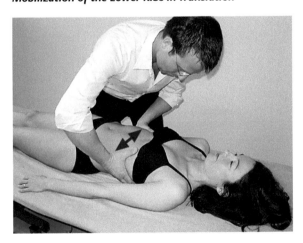

Fig. 3.18

Starting Position
The patient is in the supine position. The practitioner stands to the side of the patient.

Procedure
With both hands spread out on the right and left side, grasp the patient's lower ribs.

Treatment
Apply mobilizing pressure to the thorax in translation, alternating rhythmically to the left and to the right. This mobilization should be continued for at least 1 min.

4   Reflex Point Treatment according to Chapman

Definition

The Chapman reflex points are "gangliform contractions" in the deeper layers of the fascia. They can be described as small fascial tissue changes.

Their topographical location is relatively constant. They are associated with the internal organs.

Their location in and association with an organ are reproducible. Their existence has been substantiated by the empirical work of Chapman and Owens.

Location and Shape

The anterior reflex points are located in the intercostal spaces near the sternum. Here, we find the typical "gangliform contractions": they are about half as big as an airgun pellet or roughly the size of a bean.

The reflex points in the pelvic region can also be similarly shaped, although some are stringlike formations or unformed dispersions.

The posterior reflex points are localized along the spinal column between the spinous processes and the ends of the transverse processes. It is rare for them to assume the form of a "gangliform contraction"; they feel more edematous and transmit a stringlike palpatory sensation in deeper layers than the anterior points.

Organs have both anterior and posterior reflex points. In some cases, reflex points for an organ are found bilaterally.

Principle of Treatment

Make contact with the reflex point. For this purpose, very gently place a finger on the point and press only lightly. Reflex points are often very sensitive, so it is imperative to proceed with caution.

The finger remains on the point and treatment is by gentle rotations.

The anterior points are treated first, then the posterior points. Continue with the treatment until you have normalized the sensitivity or consistency of the point.

To conclude, check the anterior points once more. If you fail to notice any change, it is possible that the organ pathology is too great to be influenced reflexively in the short term, or other dysfunctions are present that must be treated first.

Significance of the Reflex Points

The reflex points of Chapman first of all present a diagnostic tool. To explain their operating principle, one theory states that they affect the movement of lymphatic fluid.

In addition, they are said to affect the internal organs via the vegetative nervous system.

Note
The reflex points of Chapman:
- Are a diagnostic tool
- Influence lymphatic circulation
- Influence the internal organs vegetatively

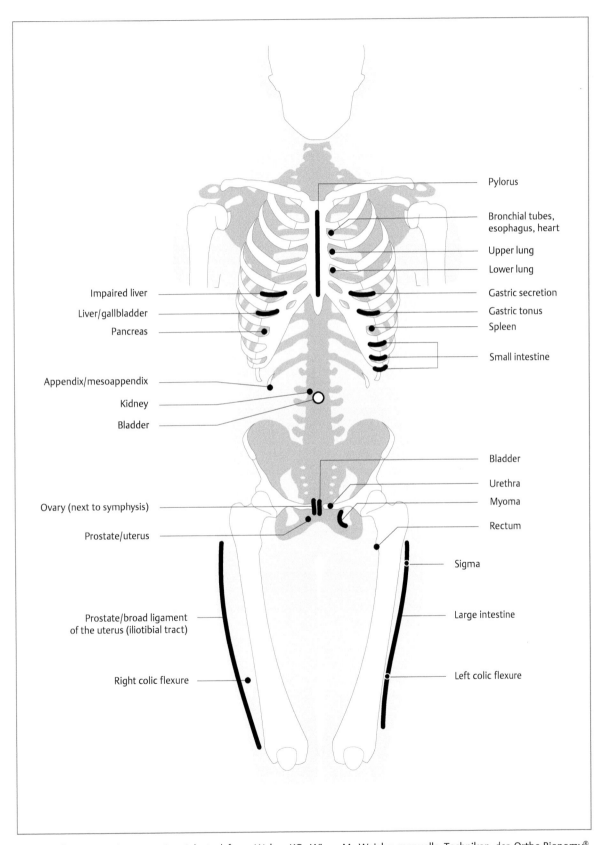

Fig. 4.1 Chapman points, anterior. Adapted from Weber KG, Wiese M. Weiche manuelle Techniken der Ortho-Bionomy®. Praktisches Lehrbuch. 2nd ed. Stuttgart: Sonntag; 2005.

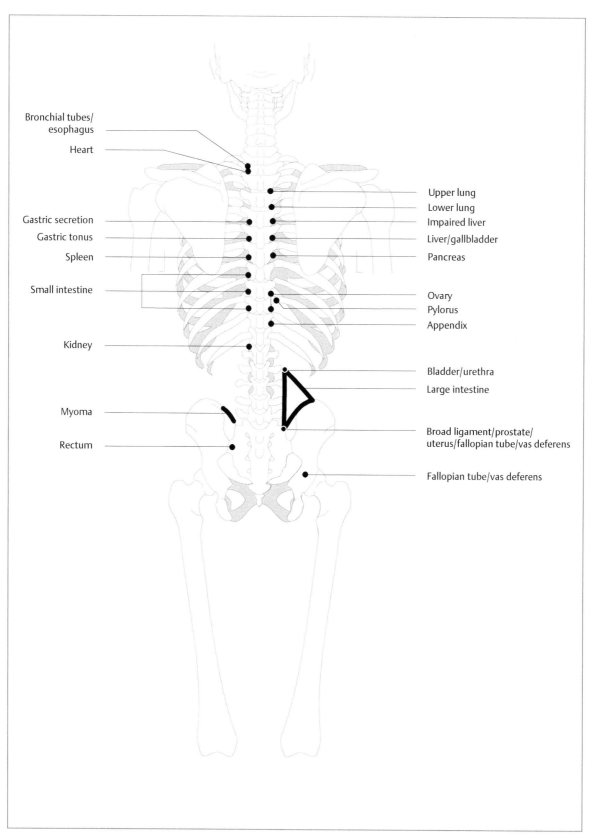

Fig. 4.2 Chapman points, posterior. Adapted from Weber KG, Wiese M. Weiche manuelle Techniken der Ortho-Bionomy®. Praktisches Lehrbuch. 2nd ed. Stuttgart: Sonntag; 2005.

II Osteopathy
of the Individual Organs

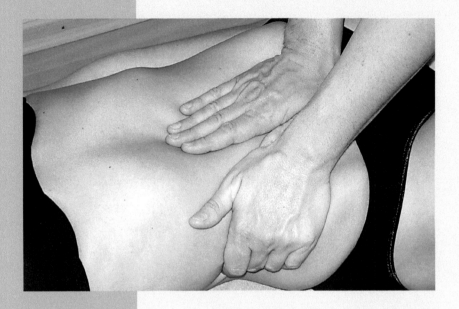

5 The Liver

Anatomy

General Facts

Macroscopic subdivision of the liver is into:
- left and right lobe
- caudate lobe
- quadrate lobe

The liver is covered by peritoneum, except for the "bare area," which is directly connected to the diaphragm. It weighs about 1.5–2.5 kg, although the effective weight is only about 400 g because the gravitational force of the thoracic organs (vacuum in the thorax), on the one hand, and the abdominal organ pressure, on the other, reduce it.

Blood flow through the liver is about 1.5 L/min.

Location

The liver is located in the right upper abdomen below the diaphragm.

Cranial Boundary

- anterior: fifth intercostal space (ICS) on the right to the sixth ICS on the left
- on the left side; extending roughly to a vertical line through the body via the center of the left inguinal ligament
- posterior: T8–T9

Caudal Boundary

- anterior: lower costal arch ascending from right to left past the center line
- posterior: T11–T12

Topographic Relationships

- dorsolateral and anterior on the right: abdominal wall and ribs 8–11
- diaphragm
- gallbladder
- hepatic/cystic/common bile duct
- inferior vena cava
- portal vein
- proper hepatic artery

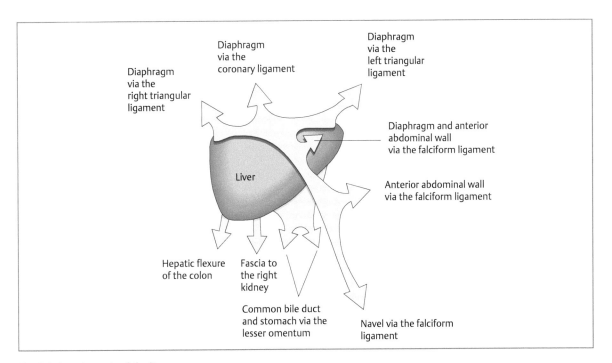

Fig. 5.1 Attachments of the liver.

- esophagus
- stomach
- right adrenal gland
- right kidney
- duodenum: superior and descending part
- right colic flexure
- indirect contact to pleura, lung, pericardium, and heart

Attachments/Suspensions

- pressure in the abdominal cavity
- turgor
- coronary ligament
- left and right triangular ligament
- falciform ligament
- round ligament of the liver
- lesser omentum (hepatoduodenal and hepatogastric ligaments)
- hepatorenal ligament
- inferior vena cava

Circulation

Arterial

Hepatic artery proper from the celiac trunk.

Venous

- portal vein (collects blood from the spleen, distal esophagus, stomach, small intestine, colon, upper rectum, pancreas, and gallbladder)
- inferior vena cava

Lymph Drainage

The lymphatic vessels run parallel to the blood vessels.

Innervation

- sympathetic nervous system from T7 to T10 via the greater and lesser splanchnic nerve
- switchover in the celiac plexus
- vagus nerve
- The liver capsule is innervated via the phrenic nerve (C3–C5).

Organ Clock

Maximal time: 1–3 a.m.
Minimal time: 1–3 p.m.

Organ–Tooth Interrelationship

Organs and teeth have a relationship to each other that is comparable to the system of connective tissue zones on the back or the foot reflex zones. Disorders or even just functional disturbances of an organ are reflected in the weakening of a tooth, the adjoining gum, or the nearby mucous membranes. The tooth can hurt without a corresponding lesion being present. Likewise, it is possible that the tooth, gums, or mucous membranes are inflamed.

Similarly, a damaged tooth also affects the corresponding organ. This can reach the point where an organic disturbance can be cured only after the tooth or gums have healed up.

For osteopaths, it is therefore important to know the interrelationships of each organ and tooth, and to take countermeasures against misdiagnoses and mistreatments early on. For this reason, the tooth associated with the organ is identified here. In this context, always remember that the adjoining gum and mucous membranes are part of this relationship as well.

- Canine tooth in the upper jaw on both sides

Movement Physiology according to Barral

Mobility

The liver displays mobility in three planes, as follows.

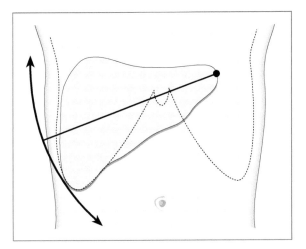

Fig. 5.2 Mobility and motility of the liver in the frontal plane.

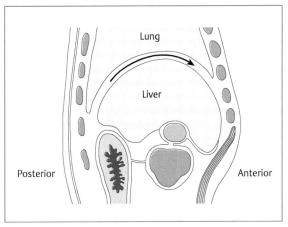

Fig. 5.3 Mobility and motility of the liver in the sagittal plane.

Frontal Plane
During inhalation, the diaphragm leads the lateral parts of the liver inferiorly to medially. Looked at from the front, the liver rotates in a counterclockwise direction.

The axis of movement is a sagittotransverse axis through the left triangular ligament.

Sagittal Plane
In this plane, the liver tilts with the cranial parts anteriorly while at the same time shifting the caudal edge posteriorly. The frontotransverse axis of movement runs approximately through the coronary ligament.

Transverse Plane
The liver carries out a leftward rotation along a fronto-sagittal axis through the inferior vena cava as an approximate anatomic landmark. Looked at from above, this is a counterclockwise rotation.

Motility

The motions of motility correspond in direction and axis to those of mobility.

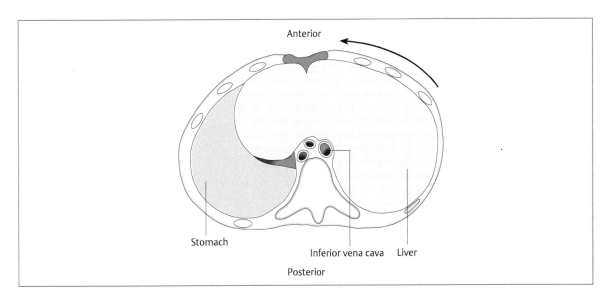

Fig. 5.4 Mobility and motility of the liver in the transverse plane.

Physiology

Metabolic Functions of the Liver

- lipolysis (metabolism of fatty acids up to coenzyme A)
- production of ketone bodies from fat, e.g., in hunger periods or in badly adjusted diabetes mellitus with bad breath smelling of acetone
- lipogenesis (production of triglycerides)
- glycogenesis and glycogenolysis
- gluconeogenesis (synthesis of glucose from lactate or amino acids)
- formation of proteins from amino acids (e.g., albumin, globulin, fibrinogen, prothrombin, vitamin K-dependent coagulation factors)
- breakdown of proteins, e.g., estrogen
- production of urea from brain—toxic ammonia, the product of protein breakdown
- breakdown and excretion of exogenous toxins, e.g., medications
- storage organ, e.g., for glycogen, or vitamin A or B_{12}
- production and excretion of bile
- synthesis and processing of cholesterol
- location of blood production up to the sixth fetal month

The liver metabolizes all three basic elements of food (carbohydrates, fats, and proteins) in different ways, therefore playing a dominant role in intermediary metabolism.

Pathologies

Symptoms that Require Medical Clarification

- Icterus
- Recurrent upper abdominal complaints
- Fever of uncertain origin
- Acute inflammation
- Cachexia

Icterus

Definition. The deposition of bilirubin causes a yellow coloration in blood plasma and connective tissue. With regard to connective tissue, the sclerae turn yellow first, followed by the skin. This phenomenon occurs when the concentration of bilirubin in the plasma exceeds 0.3–0.5 mmol/L.

Types
- **Prehepatic icterus:** the rate of erythrocyte breakdown is increased. With the liver functioning normally, the amount of accumulating hemoglobin is greater than the liver's capacity to process it. A possible cause is a congenital hemolytic anemia, e.g., thalassemia.
- **Intrahepatic icterus:** the liver cells are damaged and lose their ability to break down hemoglobin. A possible cause is acute hepatitis.

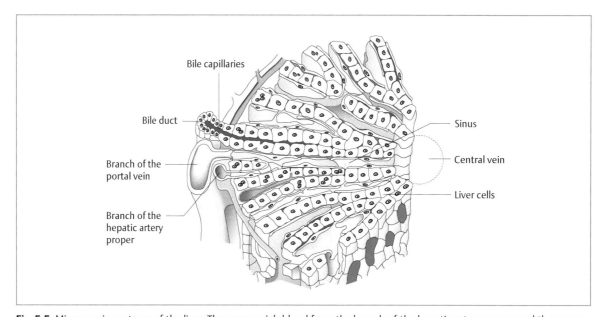

Fig. 5.5 Microscopic anatomy of the liver. The oxygen-rich blood from the branch of the hepatic artery proper and the oxygen-deficient but nutrient-rich blood from the portal vein together flow into the central vein. The numerous metabolic processes of the liver take place in the liver cells. The cells receive the necessary oxygen and "building blocks" from the mixed blood in the sinus of the liver.

- **Posthepatic icterus (obstructive icterus):** in this form of icterus, the bile ducts are compromised. They can be blocked both within the liver, e.g., in a cirrhosis, and outside the liver by a tumor or gallstones in the common bile duct. Additional causes are:
  - fatty liver
  - hepatitis
  - papillary stenosis
  - cholangitis
  - pancreatic head carcinoma
  - pancreatitis

Acute Hepatitis

Definition. Infection of the body with a pathogenic virus that affects the liver cells.

Hepatitis A

Infection. The hepatitis A virus (HAV) is most often transmitted fecally or orally, although sexual or perinatal transmission is also possible. One risk factor is traveling to southern vacation areas: even in Europe, a clear north–south divide exists in the spread of hepatitis A infection.

Clinical. The period of incubation is 14–40 days. Most frequently, we see a prodromal stage with flulike and gastrointestinal symptoms (feeling of fullness, lack of appetite, nausea, diarrhea, fever, joint pain). This is followed by the organ manifestation with icterus, sensitivity to pressure in the liver, signs of liver cell degradation, and in a fifth of all cases splenomegaly.

The course of the disease is an average of 4–8 weeks; life-long immunity remains. This type has neither virus carriers nor chronification.

Hepatitis B

Infection. In the case of the hepatitis B virus (HBV), the path of transmission is parenteral (plus needle puncture wounds), sexual contact, or perinatal. Worldwide, about 200 million people are infected.

Clinical. The period of incubation is 60–120 days. A non-specific preliminary stage can be missing; organ manifestation runs a much more serious and drawn-out course than in hepatitis A. Nevertheless, most hepatitis B infections are asymptomatic.

In 5–15% of infections, the acute form turns into the chronic form, which can lead to cirrhosis of the liver or a primary liver cell carcinoma. The disease takes a lethal course in 2–15% of all cases, but there are also healthy and infectious virus carriers.

Active immunization is advised.

Hepatitis D

Infection. The delta virus is attached to the B virus and utilizes parts of the HBV for its own reproduction. The path of infection is parenteral or by sexual contact. Endemic regions are southern Italy, the Balkans, the Near East, Africa, and South America.

Clinical. The period of incubation for simultaneous infection with HBV is 12–15 weeks. If a patient with persistent HBV is infected, the incubation period is clearly shorter, around 3 weeks.

The infection entails a serious negative effect on the liver, and not uncommonly also liver failure. Approximately 80% of hepatitis D virus (HDV) infections become chronic.

Protection against this infection is achieved by immunization against HBV.

Hepatitis C

Infection. The hepatitis C virus (HCV) is spread via injection or sexual transmission. It is found in 0.5–1.5% of all blood donors. Anti-HCV is clearly more common in people who have experienced an HBV infection.

Clinical. The period of incubation is 5–12 weeks. Asymptomatic courses are possible. Nevertheless, 50% of infections take a chronic course, and transition to cirrhosis or hepatocellular carcinoma is not uncommon.

There is no immunization.

Hepatitis E

Infection. The path of transmission for the hepatitis E virus (HEV) is fecal–oral. In developing countries, it is held responsible for epidemics of HEV infection.

Clinical. The course is identical to that of hepatitis A. There are no chronic courses or healthy virus carriers.

Women who become infected with HEV in the last trimester of pregnancy die in about 25% of cases.

Chronic Hepatitis

Definition
This condition refers to inflammatory liver disorders that persist for 6 months or longer without improvement.

Causes
- HBV infection
- HCV infection
- HDV infection
- autoimmune hepatitis
- toxins (alcohol, medications)

Clinical. We distinguish between a persistent and an aggressive type. The persistent type is marked by nonspecific symptoms such as fatigue, weight loss, and diffuse upper abdominal complaints. The prognosis is favorable.

Aggressive chronic hepatitis manifests in a disease progression with not only nonspecific symptoms but also signs of liver cirrhosis, e.g., esophageal varices.

Fatty Liver

Definition. Fatty liver refers to an increase of fat deposits in the liver cells. If more than 50% of the cells are affected, we talk about a fatty liver. If less than 50% of cells are affected, we call the condition fatty degeneration of the liver.

Causes
- alcohol abuse
- adiposity
- diabetes mellitus
- pregnancy
- toxins, e.g., poisonous mushrooms

Clinical. In most cases, hepatomegaly manifests with no complaints. The symptoms depend on the cause.

Liver Damage from Alcohol

Definition. Toxic effect on the liver as a result of excess alcohol or alcohol abuse.

Clinical
- fatty liver
- steatosis hepatitis or acute alcohol hepatitis with signs of liver insufficiency to the point of liver failure with:
  - pressure pain in the liver
  - nausea, and also weight loss
  - fever
  - icterus
  - ascites
  - hepatosplenomegaly
  - encephalopathy
- alcoholic liver cirrhosis

Cirrhosis of the Liver

Definition. Irreversible change in normal liver tissue with fibrosis and destruction of the physiologic microscopic lobe structure.

Causes
- alcohol
- HBV, HCV, HDV
- medications

- cystic fibrosis
- chronic right cardiac insufficiency

Clinical. Liver insufficiency with:
- structural tissue change: enlargement of the liver with hardening and bumpy surface (the liver shrinks terminally) and hypoperfusion of the liver
- icterus
- hepatic encephalopathy
- ascites and ankle edema (albumin deficiency)
- anemia
- a bleeding tendency

Estrogen dominance with:
- spider angioma
- men with loss of chest hair, abdominal baldness, testicular atrophy
- palmar erythema
- gynecomastia

Portal hypertension with:
- hypersplenism with bone marrow changes and pancytopenia and hemorrhagic diathesis
- splenomegaly
- esophageal varices
- caput medusae
- external hemorrhoids
- ascites

General symptoms:
- fatigue
- reduced productivity
- nonspecific upper abdominal complaints
- cachexia

Portal Hypertension

Definition. Increased pressure in the portal vein system of more than 15 mmHg.

Causes. The blood flow in the portal vein system is blocked. This obstruction in blood flow can be prehepatic, intrahepatic, or posthepatic.

Possible causes include:
- prehepatic: portal vein thrombosis
- intrahepatic: cirrhosis of the liver
- posthepatic: right cardiac insufficiency

Clinical. Development of portacaval bypass circuits with:
- esophageal varices
- caput medusae
- external hemorrhoids
- ascites (transudation of plasma fluid, e.g., via the mesenteric veins)
- splenomegaly

Primary Hepatocellular Carcinoma

Definition. This is the most common malignant liver tumor. It develops from degenerated liver cells. Make sure that you distinguish it from liver metastases of extrahepatic tumors.

Causes
- alcohol abuse
- chronic HBV and HCV
- aflatoxin poisoning (ergot alkaloids)

Clinical
- symptoms of a decompensated liver cirrhosis
- cachexia

Osteopathic Practice

Cardinal Symptoms

- Fatigue
- Icterus

Typical Dysfunctions

- adhesions/fixations
- decreased metabolic activity with loss of general vitality

Associated Structural Dysfunctions

- C0/1 and C1/2
- T7–T10
- ribs 7–10 on the right side
- C4 to T1 on the right side or bilaterally

Atypical Symptoms

Osteopathic chains often follow the fascial structures or can be explained reflexively on the basis of the vegetative innervation of the organ. As a result of the fact that the fascia is organized as an interconnected continuum of tissues, parietal or functional symptoms can arise at a great distance from the original cause (hence the dysfunction of an organ). An osteopathic chain in this context describes the anatomic–functional, often fascial, path from the cause to the symptom.

Example: hepatitis leaves behind a motor disturbance in the liver. This disturbed dynamic is transmitted via the diaphragm to the parietal pleura up to the pleural dome. To adapt to this disturbed dynamic, the cervicopleural ligaments develop nonphysiologic tissue pulls, which are transmitted to the lower cervical vertebrae. The result is a malposition of the vertebrae; the patient develops cervicobrachialgia as a parietal symptom.

With the same cause, we could also deduce a reflexive–vegetative osteopathic chain.

Recurrent vertebral blockages at T8–T9 can be attributed to a past history of hepatitis. The dysfunction in the liver leads to a sympathetic–afferent flow of information which can occur at the level of the segmental spinal cord during reflexive tonus changes in the parietal segmental skeletal muscles. The changed muscle pull causes a dysfunction in the segmentally associated vertebrae. As a result, we see blockage of these vertebrae with the corresponding symptoms (e.g., painful motor and respiratory impairment)—in the case of this example, in T8–T9, because the liver is innervated sympathetically from these segments, among others.

The following is a list of symptoms that either can be explained by means of osteopathic chains or result from the patient's history:
- restless sleep
- digestive problems in women in connection with the hormonal cycle (effect of progesterone)
- sleeping on the right side or on the abdomen is not tolerated well
- disturbed sleep and potentially waking up soaked in sweat between 1 and 3 a.m.
- pain or nausea in the right upper abdomen
- inability to tolerate certain foods, e.g., fat, coffee, alcohol, chocolate, eggs, pork, onions

In contrast to other authors, Barral additionally lists the following organ-specific symptoms:
- photophobia 1–2 hours after eating
- headache on both sides, at fixed intervals with cervicalgia or orbital pain
- chronic sinusitis
- hyperesthesia of the scalp
- bad breath smelling of acetone
- greasy skin and hair
- hair loss

Indications for Osteopathic Treatment

- adhesions
- biliary congestion
- decreased metabolic activity with reduction in general vitality, e.g., after infections
- lowered immune defense
- humeroscapular periarthritis, more likely on the right side
- ischialgia, especially on the left (with microblockage into the ascending lumbar vein and the azygos system)
- cruralgia on the right
- see also "Atypical Symptoms," above

Contraindications for Osteopathic Treatment

- icterus
- acute inflammation
- decompensated cardiac insufficiency
- Discontinue therapy if liver treatment triggers obvious vegetative reactions, e.g., strong nausea, vomiting, sweating, dizziness, tachycardia, and tendency to collapse.
- tumors of the liver or gallbladder
- palpable cervical or clavicular lymph nodes
- hepatomegaly
- splenomegaly

Notes for Clinical Application

In the author's opinion, the liver plays an eminent role in visceral manipulation. Not only is it in charge of numerous physiologic tasks surrounding the building blocks of our diet, but it also has manifold neuroanatomic and topographical relationships to other regions of the body where mostly parietal symptoms manifest, often far away from the liver; it frequently happens that the liver is responsible for these.

There are plenty of reasons why the liver appears so often in osteopathic dysfunction or is even changed pathologically. One is that there are numerous diseases that affect the liver: hepatitis A and B, infectious mononucleosis (the glandular fever of Pfeiffer), and several other viral infections are known to manifest in the liver.

In addition, the wrong diet can damage the liver (e.g., fatty liver). As the liver is the place where many exogenous and endogenous substances are broken down, it is not uncommon to find a liver that is so greatly overburdened with toxins that it can no longer function. Toxins are medications that are excreted via the liver. If a patient must regularly take medications (e.g., acetaminophen), this alone can be enough to cause a dysfunction or even structural liver damage.

Estrogens are also broken down by the liver, so orally taken hormones constitute an additional strain on the liver's metabolism.

Alcohol is the most widespread and socially accepted of all liver toxins. In people with an inherent weakness in their ability to break down alcohol naturally or with additional liver strain due to disease or medications, even a daily dose of alcohol that is generally regarded as "healthy" can lead to liver damage, and not only in the osteopathic sense. The author is convinced that a large number of the abdominal and parietal symptoms described below would never arise if the daily consumption of alcohol were clearly reduced.

The liver has a tendency to respond to any form of pathogenic strain by swelling. It is not enlarged in most cases, but can be palpated with taut resistance below the costal arch. In addition, it is clearly more sensitive to pressure than a healthy liver. If this condition becomes chronic, general symptoms follow that are not necessarily related to the liver, such as susceptibility to inflammation, stomatitis, restless sleep and loss of vitality, laryngitis, or even erectile dysfunction and weight gain due to excess estrogen. These concomitant signs all disappear as soon as the toxic load is reduced and the organ is able to recover.

In addition to general symptoms, additional parietal symptoms arise, depending on the osteopathic chain triggered by the liver.

A swollen liver can cause back pain in the area of the lumbar spinal column (LSC) on waking in the morning. The pain improves about 20 min after getting up. As the swelling impairs the flow of blood through the liver, it causes a backflow of blood into the portal vein. This description does not refer to the congestion seen in cirrhosis of the liver with ascites, caput medusae, or esophageal varices. Nevertheless, the obstruction to flow through the liver does have a hemodynamic effect, more in terms of the microcirculation or an osteopathic sense. The blood backs up through the inferior mesenteric vein into the upper rectal veins, which consequently form anastomoses with the lower rectal veins; these, in turn, connect to the internal iliac vein and ultimately to the common iliac vein. The ascending lumbar vein, which continues above the diaphragm as the azygos and hemiazygos vein, also flows into this large vein. It receives blood from the intervertebral veins, which in turn drain the internal vertebral venous plexus. The impeded flow in the liver can lead to congestion all the way back to this valveless plexus, which can then irritate the nerve roots, spinal cord, or posterior longitudinal ligament. Localized back pain, paraesthesia, or pain radiating into the legs can result. Liver congestion is particularly noticeable when lying down, because in this position the vertebral plexus can be drained only by means of respiration (and not by movement of the spinal column or leg muscle pumps). The patient therefore wakes up with back pain, which disappears a few minutes after getting up because of the additional pump mechanisms that come into action. Treatment of the liver often works "miracles" here.

Swelling of the liver causes irritation in the liver's capsule. This structure is innervated by the phrenic nerve, which transmits the afferent information cranially into the spinal cord. There, the information is processed at the segmental level and is also responded to segmentally in the form of an efferent information flow: the segmental muscles respond with hypertonicity. The following muscles are in charge of this response:
- levator scapulae
- anterior and middle scalene muscles
- subclavius
- supraspinatus
- infraspinatus
- teres major and minor
- rhomboid muscles
- deltoid muscle

- brachialis
- biceps brachii.

Hypertonicity of one or several of these muscles has a considerable impact on the biomechanics in the shoulder joint. Over time, an impingement syndrome, subdeltoid bursitis, rotator cuff tears, acromioclavicular joint arthrosis, or inflammation of the biceps tendon can develop.

Different disturbances of the cervical spinal column (CSC), interscapular pain, or pain in the superior angle of the scapula can also derive, for example, from the levator scapulae, rhomboids, or scalene muscles.

The scalene muscles and subclavius can be responsible for different circulatory syndromes in the arm: thoracic outlet syndrome, lateral and medial humeral epicondylitis, Dupuytren contracture, and Sudeck disease are grave shoulder–arm disorders that can arise from reflexive hypertonicity in the two above-mentioned muscle groups and can be treated effectively only if we also treat the liver as the cause of the complaints.

The sympathetic innervation of the liver comes from segments T7–T10. In general, the same applies here as for innervation of the liver capsule: the segmental processing of afferent stimulus streams leads to hypertonicity in the segmental muscles, which in this case refers to parts of the abdominal muscles, intercostal muscles, and autochthonic back muscles.

In patients who visit your practice with recurrent blockages always in the same vertebrae or ribs—in the case of the liver, segments T7–T10—carefully check the organs associated with these segments.

The liver is the organ that receives the entire venous blood from the gastrointestinal tract before it flows to the heart. In this way, the body makes sure that all components of food pass through the liver and can be processed there without first circulating through the whole body. This does result, however, in the problem that venous blood backs up when flow through the liver is obstructed. Grave obstructions occur in cirrhosis of the liver in the form of esophageal varices or splenomegaly. But even obstructions in flow through the liver after infections, or in the osteopathic sense as a result of disturbed mobility, can be noticeable in the organs upstream (see the earlier example of early morning back pain). In addition, the effects of liver congestion can be noticed in the stomach and small intestine. Both of these organs develop their own disturbances in tissue (from flatulence to stomach ulcers) in response to venous blood congestion.

In topographic terms, the liver is connected to many organs. If the liver has a dysfunction, and here again osteopathic liver congestion should be mentioned in particular, neighboring organs are also impacted negatively in their mobility and under certain circumstances develop pathologies. In this context, a few organs or structures are particularly likely to be affected—the kidneys, stomach, duodenum, and diaphragm. The specific effects of liver dysfunction on a particular organ are described in the relevant chapter for that organ.

Osteopathic Tests and Treatment

Direct Mobilization of the Liver

In the Frontal Plane according to Barral

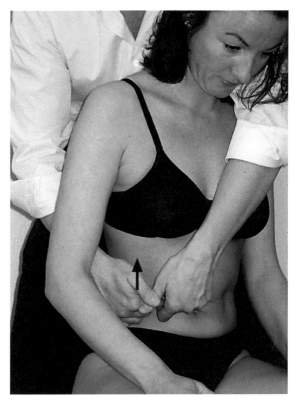

Fig. 5.6

Starting Position
The patient is sitting. The practitioner stands behind the patient.

Procedure
Place the left hand across the patient's left shoulder onto the abdominal wall on the lateral part of the right costal arch—lateral to the medioclavicular line. Pass the right hand under the patient's right armpit and place it next to the left hand.

Bring the patient into a kyphotic position. For this purpose, slide both hands simultaneously posteriorly, far below the liver.

Testing Sequence
Next, move your hands toward the underside of the liver, make contact, and evaluate the liver tissue for firmness, painfulness, and regularity of surface.

The liver should be soft, smooth, and insensitive to pressure to allow you to continue with the treatment. Under no circumstances should there be vegetative overreactions.

Now compress the liver tissue and lift the liver up cranially below the diaphragm. Release the pressure suddenly so that the liver drops back down, and evaluate the speed of its fall: if it drops slowly, more sluggishly like honey, this is an indication of low elasticity in the right triangular ligament. This ligament must show sufficient stretch to allow the liver to carry out its movement in the frontal plain without disturbance.

Treatment

For the purpose of treatment, lift the liver and let it drop again several times, as in the test. After repeating six to eight times, the speed of the fall is normalized in most cases, and the right triangular ligament is mobilized.

In the Sagittal Plane according to Barral

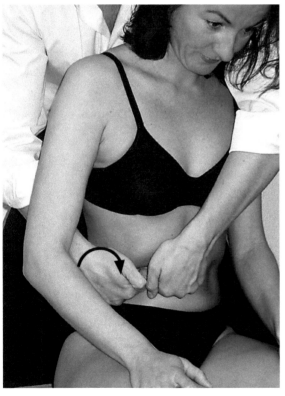

Fig. 5.7

Starting Position

The patient is sitting. The practitioner stands behind the patient.

Procedure

Pass the right hand under the patient's right armpit and place it on the abdominal wall below the right costal arch, lateral to the medioclavicular line. Pass the left hand over the patient's left shoulder and place it medial, next to the right hand, in such a way that the fingers of both hands lie next to each other below the entire right costal arch.

Bring the patient into a kyphotic position. For this purpose, slide both hands at the same time posteriorly far below the liver and finally lead both hands cranially so that the liver ends up lying in the palms of the hands.

Testing Sequence

Starting from the fingertips, initiate a tilting movement of the liver anteriorly. Release this anterior pressure suddenly and let the liver fall back posteriorly. Here again evaluate the speed of the fall. If the liver drops slowly, this indicates low elasticity in the coronary ligament. This ligament must show sufficient stretch to allow the liver to carry out its movement in the sagittal plane without disturbance.

Treatment

For the purpose of treatment, facilitate the liver and let it drop again several times, as in the test. After repeating six to eight times, the speed of the fall is normalized in most cases, and the coronary ligament is mobilized.

Indirect Mobilization of the Liver

In the Frontal Plane above the Ribs according to Barral

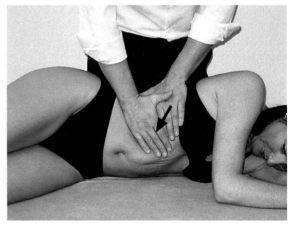

Fig. 5.8

Starting Position

The patient is lying on the left side, legs bent. The practitioner stands behind the patient.

Procedure

Place the cranial hand with the side of the little finger on top of the right lateral costal arch in the area of the rib. The caudal hand lies below the cranial hand on top of the right costal arch, but further ventrolaterally.

In a first step, press the ribs on to the liver, then mobilize the liver in a caudal–medial direction by increasing pressure on the ribs. At the end of the movement, maintain the position, initiate vibrations, or mobilize with small rebounds.

Mobilize in the opposite direction in a cranial–lateral direction in the same way.

Variation

As an alternative hand position, place one hand posteriorly and the other anteriorly on the costal arch.

In the Transverse Plane above the Ribs according to Barral

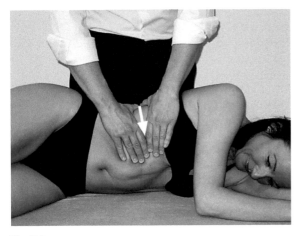

Fig. 5.9

Starting Position

The patient is lying on the left side, legs bent. The practitioner stands behind the patient.

Procedure

Place the cranial hand with the side of the little finger on top of the right lateral costal arch in the area of the fifth/sixth rib. The fingers point anteriorly and the thumb posteriorly. The caudal hand lies below the cranial hand on the right costal arch in the same way. In a first step, press the ribs onto the liver, then mobilize the liver into a leftward rotation (seen from above as a counterclockwise rotation) by increasing pressure on the ribs. At the end of the movement, maintain the position, initiate vibrations, or mobilize with small rebounds.

Similarly, mobilize into a rightward rotation in the opposite direction, but with a clearly reduced range of motion.

Variation

As an alternative hand position, place one hand posteriorly and the other hand anteriorly on the costal arch.

In the Sagittal Plane above the Ribs according to Barral

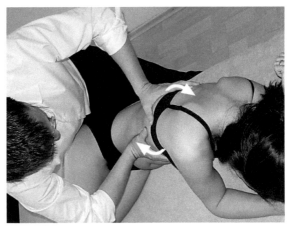

Fig. 5.10

Starting Position

The patient is lying on the left side, legs bent. The practitioner stands behind the patient.

Procedure

Place the cranial hand on the right costal arch posteriorly at the level of the fifth/sixth rib, and the caudal hand anteriorly on the right costal arch with the side of the little finger on the lower edge of the costal arch. In a first step, press the ribs onto the liver. Now use both hands to mobilize the liver in the sagittal plane by pushing the liver across the ribs anterosuperiorly with the cranial hand and posteroinferiorly with the caudal hand. At the end of the movement, maintain the position, initiate vibrations, or mobilize with small rebounds.

In the same way, mobilize the opposite direction, but with a clearly reduced range of motion.

In the Frontal Plane with Long Arm Lever according to Barral

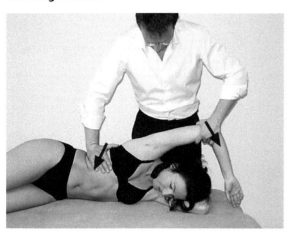

Fig. 5.11

Starting Position
The patient is lying on the left side, legs bent. The practitioner stands behind the patient.

Procedure
Place the caudal hand on the right costal arch ventrolaterally across the liver, with the fingertips pointing anteriorly.

The cranial hand takes hold of the patient's right hand and guides it into abduction until the movement arrives at the costal arch.

The caudal hand is the fixed point. The cranial hand mobilizes the liver in the frontal plane by intensifying the arm abduction. At the end of the movement, maintain the position, initiate vibrations, or mobilize in small rebounds with the caudal hand.

In this way, you improve mobility in the gliding surface between liver and diaphragm.

Variation
Alternatively, you can exchange the fixed point and the moving point, or use both levers as moving points.

You can also choose the supine position as the starting position.

In the Frontal Plane with Long Leg Lever according to Barral

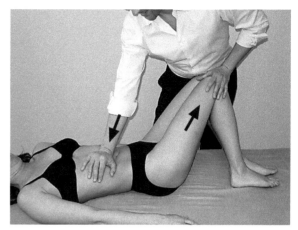

Fig. 5.12

Starting Position
The patient is in the supine position, legs bent. The practitioner stands on the patient's left side.

Procedure
Place the cranial hand with the thenar below the right costal arch and use it to push in the cranial–lateral direction. The caudal hand takes hold of the patient's right knee.

The cranial hand mobilizes the liver in the cranial–lateral direction, while the caudal hand pulls both knees to the left until the movement reaches the cranial hand. At the end of the movement, apply a continuous or intermittent pull to the structures. Both hands are moving points.

The mobilizing effect has an effect on the gliding surfaces of the liver with their caudal visceral joints.

Variation
You can also make one hand the fixed point and the other the moving point.

Liver Pump according to Barral

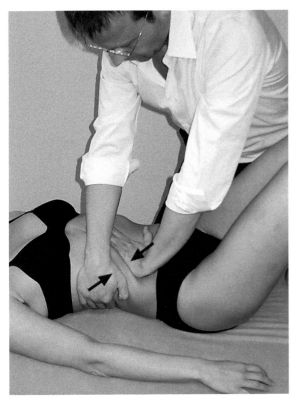

Fig. 5.13

Oscillations on the Liver

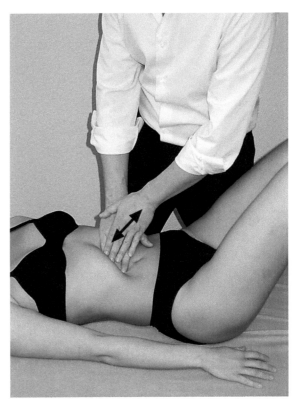

Fig. 5.14

Starting Position
The patient is in the supine position, legs bent. The practitioner stands on the patient's left side.

Procedure
With the cranial hand, enfold the right costal arch in such a way that the fingers end up lying posteriorly and the thenar laterally. Place the caudal hand with the side of the little finger below the costal arch.

During the patient's exhalation, the caudal hand pushes in the direction of the right shoulder while at the same time the cranial hand pulls the costal arch toward the caudal hand. In this way, the liver is compressed. During inhalation, maintain the position reached, and increase it further during the next exhalation.

Repeat this through two or three breaths. Then ask the patient to inhale deeply and, during the start of this inhalation, release the pressure with both hands simultaneously and abruptly.

Variation
You can also place the caudal hand with the thenar below the costal arch.

Starting Position
The patient is in the supine position, legs bent. The practitioner stands on the patient's left side.

Procedure
Place the right hand with the side of the little finger below the costal arch; place the left hand on top of it. With both hands, apply light and intermittent pressure to the liver with a frequency of 150–180/min. Maintain these oscillations for about 2 min.

This technique has a good circulatory effect.

Test and Treatment of Liver Motility
according to Barral

Fascial Treatment according to
Finet and Williame

Global Technique

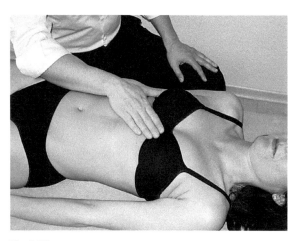

Fig. 5.15

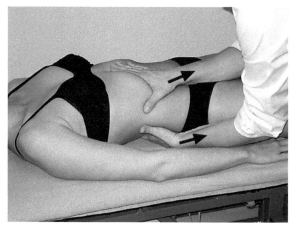

Fig. 5.16

Starting Position
The patient is in the supine position, legs stretched out. The practitioner sits by the patient's right side, facing the head.

Procedure
Place the right hand without pressure on the patient's abdomen. The thenar lies on the right lower ribs above the liver, and the fingertips rest on the left side of the thorax in the area of the left triangular ligament. The forearm rests on the abdomen.

Testing Sequence
Detect the motility movement. Evaluate the amplitude and direction of the inspiration and expiration movements as well as the rhythm of the movement as a whole. If a disturbance is present in one or both aspects of the motility movement, treat the patient.

Treatment
Motility is treated indirectly by following the unimpaired movement, remaining at the end-point of this movement for several cycles, and then following the impaired movement to the new end-point.

You can also try to increase the free movement in its range (induction). Subsequently, check whether the impaired movement direction has improved.

Repeat this movement again and again until the motility has returned to normal in terms of rhythm, direction, and amplitude.

It is best to detect the motility movement in the frontal plane.

Starting Position
The patient is in the supine position, legs stretched out. The practitioner stands by the patient's right side.

Procedure
Place the right hand anteriorly immediately below the right costal arch, with the side of the radial index finger on the lower edge of the costal arch. Place the left hand posteriorly on the ribs at the same height as the anterior hand.

With the right hand, apply pressure posteriorly until you reach the fascial plane.

Treatment
During inhalation, both hands simultaneously pull caudally. During exhalation, maintain the reached position. Repeat this procedure until you have reached the end of the fascial movement. Release the pull in the next exhalation.

Repeat the whole treatment four or five times.

Lobus Technique

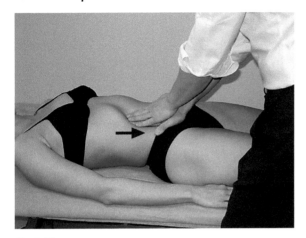

Fig. 5.17

Starting Position

The patient is in the supine position, legs stretched out. The practitioner stands by the patient's right side.

Procedure

Place both hands on top of each other on the abdomen below the right costal arch:

- in the area of the Murphy point
- medial to this
- lateral to this

The fingertips point cranially. With both hands, apply pressure posteriorly until you reach the fascial plane.

Treatment

During inhalation, both hands simultaneously pull caudally. During exhalation, maintain the position reached. Repeat this procedure until you have reached the end of the fascial movement. In the next exhalation, release the pull.

Repeat the whole treatment four or five times.

Circulatory Techniques according to Kuchera

Arterial Stimulation

- stimulation of the celiac trunk by working on the spinal column
- diaphragm techniques

Venous Stimulation

- liver pump
- stretching the hepatoduodenal ligament
- diaphragm techniques

Lymphatic Stimulation

- lymph drainage on thorax and abdomen
- diaphragm techniques

Vegetative Harmonization

Sympathetic nervous system:
Stimulation of the sympathetic trunk T7–T10 by:

- rib raising
- inhibiting the paravertebral muscles
- vibrations
- manipulations
- Maitland technique
- stimulation of the celiac plexus
- diaphragm techniques

Parasympathetic nervous system:
Stimulation of the vagus nerve by:

- craniosacral therapy
- laryngeal techniques
- thoracic techniques (recoil)
- diaphragm techniques

Reflex Point Treatment according to Chapman

Location

Liver

Anterior. Intercostal space between the sixth and seventh ribs, from parasternal to lateral to approximately the level of the mamillary line; present only on the right side!

Posterior. Between the two transverse processes T6–T7, halfway between the spinous process and the tip of the transverse process; present only on the right side!

Liver Deficiency

Anterior. Intercostal space between the fifth and sixth ribs, from parasternal to lateral to approximately the level of the mamillary line; present only on the right side!

Posterior. Between the two transverse processes of T5–T6, halfway between the spinous process and the tip of the transverse process; present only on the right side!

Treatment Principle

Make contact with the reflex point. For this purpose, very gently place a finger on the point and exert only light pressure. Reflex points are often very sensitive, and it is therefore imperative to proceed with caution.

The finger remains on the point and treatment is by gentle rotations.

The anterior points are treated first, then the posterior points. Continue with the treatment until you have normalized the sensitivity or consistency of the point.

To conclude, check the anterior points once more. If you fail to notice any change, it is possible that the organ pathology is too great to be influenced quickly via the reflex points, or other dysfunctions are present that must be treated first.

Recommendations for the Patient

- Avoid foods that contain sulfur, which can affect the performance of the liver and gallbladder, e. g., potato chips, fast foods, canned mushrooms, preserved foods.
- Avoid foods that trigger problems.
- Liver cleanse: every day (continuing for at least 14 days), take the following:
  - the juice of one lemon and a tablespoon of cold-pressed olive oil with a little water
  - bitter greens
  - liver compress with hot moist towels
  - 2–3 L of fluid a day

6　The Gallbladder

Anatomy

General Facts

The gallbladder is a hollow pear-shaped organ that measures 8–12 cm in length and 4–5 cm in width. Its capacity lies around 40–70 mL; it is the storage organ for the bile.

It is divided into:

- the fundus
- the body
- the neck

The hepatic duct (drainage path from the liver for the bile) and cystic duct (drainage path from the gallbladder) combine to form the common bile duct, which via the ampulla of Vater (major duodenal papilla) leads to the descending part of the duodenum.

The hepatic duct is 3–4 cm long and measures 3–4 mm in diameter. The common bile duct is about 6 cm long and measures 5–6 mm in diameter. At the mouth it narrows to about half this.

The mucous membrane of the neck of the gallbladder is folded into spirally shaped creases. This prevents an uncontrolled excretion of bile.

Location

The gallbladder is located intraperitoneally on the posterior side of the liver.

The axis of the gallbladder runs from caudal, anterior right, to cranial, posterior left.

Projection onto the Wall of the Torso

The fundus of the gallbladder is found at the Murphy point: draw a line connecting the navel to the right nipple or the medioclavicular point on the right. The fundus of the gallbladder can be palpated at the point where this line crosses the lower costal arch on the right. In children, this point is located further medially.

The cystic duct and hepatic duct combine to form the common bile duct in the hepatoduodenal ligament at the height of the lower edge of L1. The common bile duct lies about 10–15 cm below the anterior torso wall.

Its initial part still runs inside the ligament, i.e., intraperitoneally. At the upper edge of the superior part of the duodenum, it crosses to the posterior side of the duodenum; here its location becomes retroperitoneal. It forms an arch to the right, crosses the head of the pancreas, enters the descending part of the duodenum from posteriorly, and ends at the major duodenal papilla at approximately the height of L3. It forms a crease that is about 2 cm long on the posterior side of the descending part before it ends there.

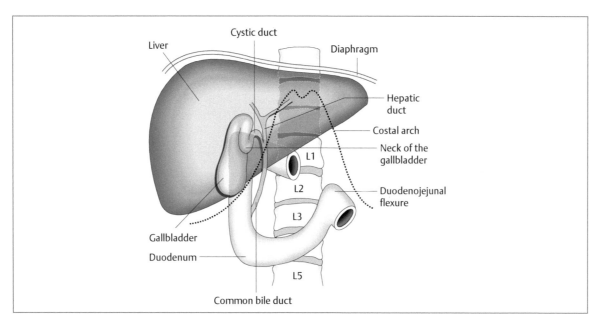

Fig. 6.1 Location of the gallbladder.

Topographic Relationships

Gallbladder

- liver
- duodenum
- greater omentum
- lesser omentum
- peritoneum

Common Bile Duct

- hepatoduodenal ligament
- proper hepatic artery
- portal vein
- posterior side of the superior part of the duodenum
- pancreas
- major duodenal papilla and descending part of the duodenum
- inferior vena cava

Attachments/Suspensions

- turgor
- organ pressure
- connection to the liver via connective tissue

Circulation

Arterial

Cystic artery (from the proper hepatic artery).

Venous

Cystic vein (to portal vein).

Innervation

- sympathetic nervous system from T7 to T10 via the greater and lesser splanchnic nerve
- switchover in the celiac plexus
- vagus nerve
- phrenic nerve, sensory branch

Organ Clock

Maximal time: 11 p.m.–1 a.m.
Minimal time: 11 a.m.–1 p.m.

Organ–Tooth Interrelationship

For basic information, see page 34.

> - Canine tooth in the lower jaw on both sides

Movement Physiology according to Barral

Mobility

In its mobility, the gallbladder is coupled to the mobility of the liver. We do not find any separate mobility.

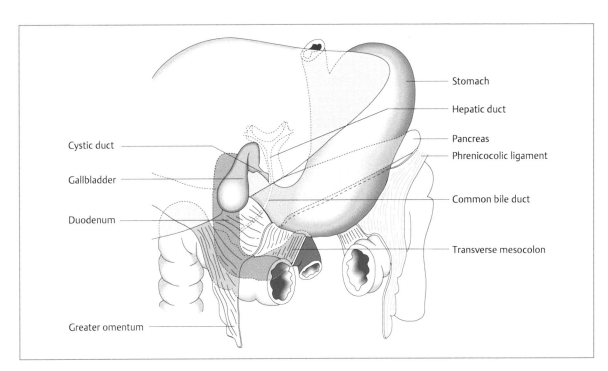

Cystic duct

Gallbladder

Duodenum

Greater omentum

Stomach

Hepatic duct

Pancreas

Phrenicocolic ligament

Common bile duct

Transverse mesocolon

Fig. 6.2 Topographic relationships of the gallbladder.

Motility

The common bile duct performs an S-shaped movement: during exhalation, we first detect a movement in a posterior–medial and then in an anterior–lateral direction; during inhalation, it is in the opposite direction.

The gallbladder is motorically coupled to the liver.

Physiology

The liver produces 800–1000 mL of bile per day. This bile is concentrated 10- to 12-fold in the gallbladder by removing water and electrolytes stored there.

Composition of Bile in the Gallbladder

- water and salt in isotonic proportions; the pH value is neutral to lightly alkaline
- phlegm
- bile pigments (bilirubin; also in small amounts biliverdin)
- bile salts
- cholesterol
- steroid medications and other foreign substances

The **bile salts** are produced in the liver from cholesterol and the amino acids glycine and taurine. They activate lipase in the small intestine and pancreas and, as separate molecules, possess hydrophilic (amino acids) and lipophilic (cholesterol) sides. In the intestinal lumen, the bile salts combine with the products of lipolysis (glycerin and fatty acids) to form **micelles**. In this form, the fatty acids, which have a low solubility in water, can be emulsified in the watery environment of the intestines and absorbed by the mucous membranes of the small intestine.

In the terminal ileum, the bile salts are reabsorbed, transported back to the liver, and again excreted into the bile (enterohepatic cycle). A bile salt molecule runs through this cycle about 18 times.

If bile salts are not reabsorbed in the ileum, they increase the water permeability of the epithelium in the colon (chologenic diarrhea).

Bilirubin is a product of the breakdown of hemoglobin from the erythrocytes. Hemoglobin is broken down in the liver into water-soluble bilirubin (conjugated with glucuronic acid) and excreted into the bile.

In the intestines, bilirubin is broken down by bacteria through several intermediate stages to urobilin and stercobilin. These end-products are responsible for the normal coloration of stools. If the passage through the intestines is too quick, the bacteria do not have enough time to break the bilirubin down completely—the stool is yellow.

In cases of cholestasis, bilirubin is lacking in the intestines and the stool is gray.

Some of the bilirubin and its metabolites are introduced into an enterohepatic cycle and finally excreted with the urine. This is the reason for the typical yellow color of urine.

The **secretion of bile** from the liver is steered by concentration of bile salts in the blood plasma—insulin, glucagon, secretin, and cholecystokinin (CCK).

The vagus nerve, secretin, gastrin, and CCK direct the voiding of the gallbladder. CCK is the strongest stimulus for the gallbladder's contraction: when mashed food arrives in the duodenum, it is stretched. As a result, CCK is secreted into the blood, and a parasympathetic stimulus causes the muscular contraction of the gallbladder, which leads to voiding. At the sphincter of Oddi, the parasympathetic stimulus causes a drop in tonicity—the sphincter opens.

However, the flow of bile from the gallbladder starts even before the food arrives in the stomach: peristalsis in the esophagus reflexively triggers the contraction of the gallbladder and relaxation of the sphincter of Oddi (enteroenteral reflex).

The **direction of bile flow** into the gallbladder or duodenum is guided by the pressure conditions in the sphincter of Oddi, bile ducts, and the gallbladder.

During the interdigestive phase, the sphincter of Oddi is closed and the pressure there is greater than in the bile ducts and gallbladder. As a result, the bile that is secreted in the liver flows through the cystic duct into the gallbladder.

Gallbladder contractions cause the pressure in the gallbladder to rise to the point where it surpasses the pressure in the sphincter. Bile from the liver and gallbladder flows into the intestines. In addition, the hormonally guided gallbladder contractions also lower tonicity in the sphincter of Oddi—so the pressure there drops at the same time as the gallbladder is voided.

The ampulla of Vater also runs into the pancreatic duct. Normally, the pressure in this duct is so great that bile juices cannot flow into the pancreas. When the ampulla is blocked, e.g., by a gallstone, this can cause the flow of bile to reverse in the direction of the pancreas.

Pathologies

Symptoms that Require Medical Clarification

- Positive Murphy sign
- Icterus
- Colic pain in the right upper abdomen

Cholelithiasis

Definition. Formation of cholesterol, pigment, or calcium stones in the gallbladder, or intra- or extrahepatic bile ducts; 99% of these stones are cholesterol stones.

Causes. Predisposing factors include:
- diabetes mellitus
- cirrhosis of the liver
- diseases of the terminal ileum
- pregnancy
- oral contraceptives

Clinical. Approximately 50% of cases run their course silently. There is abnormal, right-sided, upper abdominal pain after eating.

If a stone is stuck in the bile ducts, colic pain in the right upper abdomen radiates into the right shoulder.

Cholecystitis

Definition. Inflammation of the wall of the gallbladder, most commonly the result of cholelithiasis.

Causes
- impacted stones
- invasion by intestinal germs

Clinical
- nausea
- vomiting
- fever
- scleral icterus
- positive Murphy sign

Gallbladder Carcinoma

Definition. In most cases, we are dealing with adenocarcinomas.

Causes
- cholelithiasis (in 95% of diseases, this is the previous medical history)
- adenomas of the gallbladder

Clinical
- obstructive icterus

Osteopathic Practice

Cardinal Symptom

- Positive Murphy sign

Typical Dysfunctions

- adhesions/fixations
- spasms

Associated Structural Dysfunctions

- C0/1 and C1/2
- C4–C6, more commonly on the left
- ribs 7–10 on the right side

Atypical Symptoms

The following is a list of symptoms that can be explained by means of osteopathic chains or result from the patient's history (for an explanation of osteopathic chains, see "Atypical Symptoms" in Chapter 5, page 39):
- humeroscapular periarthritis, possibly on both sides
- cervicalgia
- pain is interscapular or by the superior scapular angle on the right
- hyperesthetic zone on the back: T12 on the right paravertebra (Boas sign)
- low tolerance for prone position
- disturbed sleep and waking up between 11 p.m. and 1 a.m. soaked in sweat
- inability to tolerate certain foods, e.g., fat, coffee, alcohol, chocolate, eggs, pork, onions

In contrast to other authors, Barral additionally lists the following organ-specific symptoms:
- in women: complaints increase in the second half of the menstrual cycle (effect of progesterone)
- headache, beginning left frontal
- eye pain on the left
- hypersensitive scalp on the left side
- preference for certain foods, e.g., vinegar, pepper, mustard

Indications for Osteopathic Treatment

Disturbed bile secretion with dyssynergia of gallbladder, bile ducts, and sphincter of Oddi. Causes for this problem can be adhesions, spasms, or in women menstrual factors (see also "Atypical Symptoms" above).

Contraindications for Osteopathic Treatment

- icterus
- biliary colic
- cholecystitis
- tumors of the liver, gallbladder, bile ducts, and pancreas

Gallstones can become dislodged and trigger colic, but do not present a contraindication as such.

If a gallbladder treatment triggers obvious vegetative reactions, e.g., severe nausea, vomiting, sweating, dizziness, tendency to collapse, and tachycardia, stop the treatment.

Osteopathic Tests and Treatment

Murphy Sign

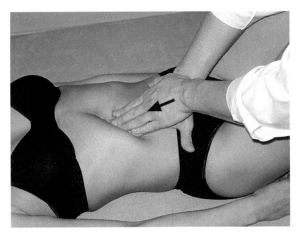

Fig. 6.3

Starting Position
The patient is in the supine position. The practitioner stands by the patient's right side.

Procedure
Push your right hand under the right costal arch in the area of the gallbladder. If you can trigger obvious pressure pain during deep inhalations (watch facial expression) and the patient stops inhaling, Murphy sign is positive.

This is a sign of a gallbladder pathology that requires clarification by a physician.

Treatment of the Sphincter of Oddi (Major Duodenal Papilla) according to Barral

To improve the flow of bile, begin by treating the sphincter of Oddi, which frees drainage.

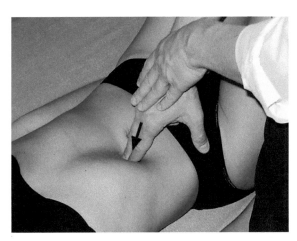

Fig. 6.4

Starting Position
The patient is in the supine position, legs bent. The practitioner stands on the patient's right side.

Procedure
To find the sphincter of Oddi, you have to determine its approximate projection onto the abdominal wall. For this purpose, move from the navel about three finger-widths cranially. From there, move horizontally in a lateral direction until you cross a line that connects the navel and the right nipple (or the navel and the intersection between the right medioclavicular line and the right costal arch). At this point, slowly slide posteriorly into the abdomen. It is important here to proceed slowly, so that the superficial intestinal loops and the transverse colon have enough time to move away from the pressure and the fascia can relax.

Once you have advanced deeply enough in this palpation, you will usually find a supple, roughly pea-sized solidification within 0.5–1 cm of this palpation point. In most cases, the sphincter is sensitive to palpation.

You can now carry out small circulations, vibrations, or inhibitions on this point, until the tonus or soreness is clearly reduced.

Voiding the Gallbladder in Seated Position according to Barral

Smoothing Out and Stretching the Biliary Tract according to Barral

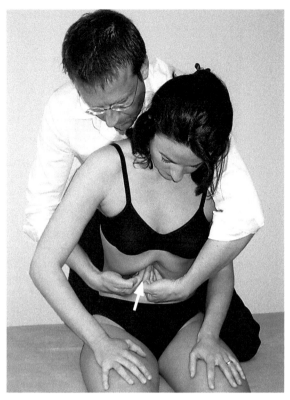

Fig. 6.5

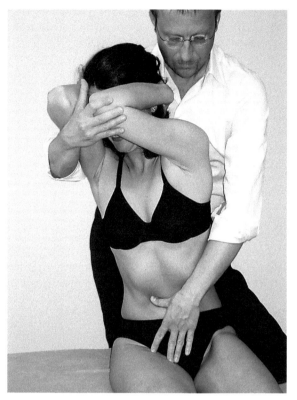

Fig. 6.6

Starting Position

The patient is sitting. The practitioner stands behind the patient.

Procedure

Guide your left hand over the patient's left shoulder onto the abdominal wall at the palpation point of the gallbladder (Murphy point) below the right costal arch. Pass the right hand under the patient's right armpit and place it next to the left hand.

Bring the patient into a kyphotic position by sliding both hands simultaneously in a posterior–cranial–left direction onto the fundus of the gallbladder.

Now press the organ gently cranially against the liver. Then continue moving both hands along the axis of the gallbladder in a posterior–cranial–left direction and repeat this procedure at a different point on the body of the gallbladder. Proceed in this way up to the neck of the gallbladder.

Variation

Instead of releasing the pressure on the gallbladder again and again, you can also smooth out the organ with a continuous pull to its neck. This technique resembles squeezing out a tube of toothpaste from the back to the front.

Starting Position

The patient is sitting, hands clasped to the neck and elbows pointing forward. The practitioner stands behind the patient.

Procedure

The technique is performed as described above. When you have arrived at the neck of the gallbladder, replace the palpation fingers with the two thumbs and stroke along a line parallel to the median line but slightly to its right, in a caudal direction. At the upper edge of the superior part of the duodenum, change the stroking direction: guide the thumbs in a rightward arch to the major duodenal papilla.

Now use the left thumb to fix the common bile duct on the papilla, while you grasp both of the patient's elbows with the right hand and facilitate an extension, rightward rotation, and lateral flexion to the left.

This movement sets off a stretch impulse in the biliary tract.

The common bile duct is not palpated directly in this technique. Instead, the desired effect is obtained by compressing the more anteriorly lying structures on the tract.

Stretching the Biliary Tract by Lifting the Liver

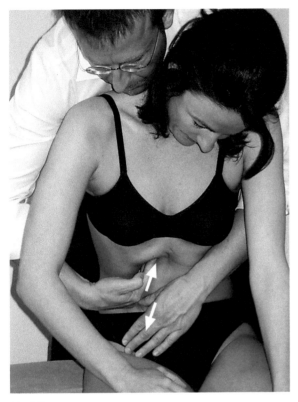

Fig. 6.7

Starting Position
The patient is sitting. The practitioner stands behind the patient.

Procedure
Pass your hands under the patient's armpits to the palpation point of the gallbladder (Murphy point) below the right costal arch.

Bring the patient into a kyphotic position by sliding both hands simultaneously in a posterior–cranial–left direction onto the fundus of the gallbladder. Now palpate forward up to the neck of the gallbladder and stabilize it with your right hand. With the left hand, palpate along the biliary tract caudally until you reach the sphincter of Oddi (see page 53) and fix the common bile duct at this point.

With the right hand, press the neck of the gallbladder in a cranial direction and lift the liver up; with the left hand press the fixed point caudally. As a result, the biliary tract is stretched.

Smoothing Out and Stretching the Common Bile Duct in Supine Position according to Barral

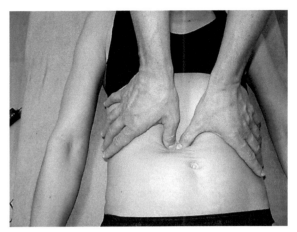

Fig. 6.8

Starting Position
The patient is in the supine position. The practitioner stands at the head of the table.

Procedure
Place both thumbs or the hypothenar of one hand on the abdomen on top of the projection of the upper edge of the superior duodenum (slightly to the right of the pylorus, see page 73). Compress the tissue on the common bile duct and smooth out the common bile duct in a rightward arch to the ampulla of Vater.

De-spasming the Gallbladder according to Barral

Starting Position
The patient is sitting. The practitioner stands behind the patient.

Procedure (see Fig. 6.5)
Guide your left hand over the patient's left shoulder onto the abdominal wall at the palpation point of the gallbladder (Murphy point) below the right costal arch. Pass the right hand under the patient's right armpit and place it next to the left hand.

Bring the patient into a kyphotic position by sliding both hands simultaneously in a posterior–cranial–left direction onto the fundus of the gallbladder.

A spasmed location is more painful than the rest of the gallbladder and also shows a higher tonicity. When you have found such a place, gently press it cranially against the liver and then abruptly release this pressure in a rebound. Repeat this until the spasm is released.

Then continue moving both hands a little further along the axis of the gallbladder in a posterior–cranial–

left direction and repeat this procedure at a different spasmed point on the body of the gallbladder.

Defibrosing the Gallbladder according to Barral

Starting Position
The patient is sitting. The practitioner stands behind the patient.

Procedure (see Fig. 6.5)
A fibrosed location is clearly indurated, e.g., as a consequence of surgery or inflammation, but not necessarily painful.

Guide your left hand over the patient's left shoulder onto the abdominal wall at the palpation point of the gallbladder (Murphy point) below the right costal arch. Pass the right hand under the patient's right armpit and place it next to the left hand.

Bring the patient into a kyphotic position by sliding both hands simultaneously in a posterior–cranial–left direction onto the fundus of the gallbladder.

Palpate the fibrosed location, press it against the liver, and help the patient achieve a rotation around this fixed point. The rotation mobilizes the fibrosis, which is clearly noticeable as a relaxation of the tissue. Proceed in this manner with each area of fibrosed wall.

Oscillations on the Murphy Point

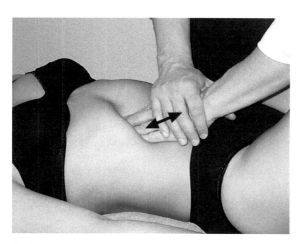

Fig. 6.9

Starting Position
The patient is in the supine position, legs bent. The practitioner stands on the patient's left side.

Procedure
Gently guide the fingers of the right hand under the costal arch at the Murphy point. At the fundus of the gallbladder, apply oscillations, i.e., press lightly and intermit-

tently on the fundus with a frequency of 150–180/min. Continue these oscillations for about 2 min.

This technique results in a healthy decrease in tonicity and supports voiding of the gallbladder. It should be utilized when direct treatment under the costal arch in the seated position is not tolerated.

Test and Treatment of Motility in the Common Bile Duct according to Barral

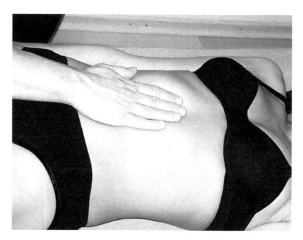

Fig. 6.10

Starting Position
The patient is in the supine position, legs stretched out. The practitioner sits by the patient's right side, facing the head.

Procedure
Without applying pressure, place the thenar of your right hand on the patient's abdomen immediately below the right costal arch at the umbilico-medioclavicular line. The fingers point cranially, the forearm rests on the abdomen.

Testing Sequence
Detect the motility movement as described above and evaluate the amplitude and direction of the inspiratory and expiratory movements as well as the rhythm of the movement as a whole. If a disturbance is present in one or both aspects of the motility movement, treat the patient.

Treatment
Motility is treated indirectly by following the unimpaired movement, remaining at the end-point of this movement for several cycles, and then following the impaired movement to the new end-point.

You can also try to increase the range of the free movement (induction), afterward checking whether the limited movement direction has improved.

Repeat this movement again and again until the motility has returned to normal in terms of rhythm, direction, and amplitude.

Fascial Treatment according to Finet and Williame

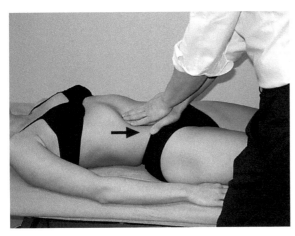

Fig. 6.11

Starting Position
The patient is in the supine position, legs stretched out. The practitioner stands next to the patient.

Procedure
Place both hands on top of each other on the abdomen below the right costal arch in the area of the Murphy point. With both hands, apply just enough pressure posteriorly to reach the fascial plane.

Treatment
During inhalation, both hands simultaneously pull caudally. During expiration, maintain the reached position. Repeat this procedure until you have reached the end of the fascial movement. In the next exhalation, release the pull.
Repeat the whole treatment four or five times.

Circulatory Techniques according to Kuchera

Arterial Stimulation
- stimulation of the celiac trunk by working on the spinal column
- diaphragm techniques

Venous Stimulation
- liver pump
- stretching the hepatoduodenal ligament
- diaphragm techniques

Lymphatic Stimulation
- lymph drainage on thorax and abdomen
- diaphragm techniques

Vegetative Harmonization
Sympathetic nervous system:
Stimulation of the sympathetic trunk T7–T10 by:
- rib raising
- inhibiting the paravertebral muscles
- vibrations
- manipulations
- Maitland technique
- stimulation of the celiac plexus
- diaphragm techniques

Parasympathetic nervous system:
Stimulation of the vagus nerve by:
- craniosacral therapy
- laryngeal techniques
- thoracic techniques (recoil)
- diaphragm techniques

Reflex Point Treatment according to Chapman

Location

Anterior. Intercostal space between sixth and seventh ribs, from parasternal to lateral approximately to the level of the mamillary line; present only on the right side!

Posterior. Between the two transverse processes of T6 and T7, halfway between the spinous process and the tip of the transverse process; present only on the right side!

Treatment Principle
Make contact with the reflex point. For this purpose, very gently place a finger on the point and press only lightly. Reflex points are often very sensitive, so it is imperative to proceed with caution.
    The finger remains on the point and treatment is by gentle rotations.
    The anterior points are treated first, then the posterior points. Continue with the treatment until you have normalized the sensitivity or consistency of the point.
    To conclude, check the anterior points once more. If you fail to notice any change, it is possible that the organ pathology is too great to be influenced quickly via the reflex points, or other dysfunctions are present that must be treated first.

Recommendations for the Patient

- Gallbladder treatments can trigger epigastric pain or nausea to the point of vomiting. Normally, these symptoms disappear after a few days. Make your patients aware of this fact.
- Avoid foods that trigger discomfort.
- Avoid foods that contain sulfur, which can affect the performance of the liver and gallbladder, e.g., potato chips, fast food, canned mushrooms, preserved foods.
- Being overweight increases the risk of gallstones.
- Regularly eat mussels, tuna, and lamb (rich in taurine).

7 The Stomach

Anatomy

▥ Anatomy of the Esophagus

Location

The esophagus is located in the posterior mediastinum. It lies medial in front of the spinal column until the tracheal bifurcation (T4), after which it moves to the right side, to make room for the heart. Lastly, it crosses the diaphragm to the left of the median line. At the level of T7–T8, the aorta squeezes in between the spinal column and the esophagus. The abdominal part is only about 2 cm long.

Topographic Relationships

Thorax

- trachea
- left main bronchus
- mediastinal pleura
- pericardium
- spinal column
- aorta
- right lung (in the area of the esophageal hiatus)
- vagus nerve, right and left

Abdomen

- peritoneum in the front
- liver
- crus to the left of the diaphragm
- left side: left triangular ligament
- right side: lesser omentum
- T10 and T11

Attachments/Suspensions

- organ pressure
- turgor
- mediastinal connective tissue
- phrenoesophageal ligament (ring-shaped disk in the hiatus).

The esophagus remains mobile in the lengthwise direction.

Circulation

Cervical

- inferior thyroid artery
- small branches from the subclavian/communal carotid/vertebral arteries, etc.
- inferior thyroid vein (from the superior vena cava)

Thoracic

- bronchial arteries
- aorta
- azygos/hemiazygos/accessory hemiazygos vein (from the superior vena cava)

Abdominal

- left gastric artery
- inferior phrenic artery
- celiac trunk
- left gastric vein (main drainage) to the portal vein

Lymph Drainage

- deep cervical cord (internal jugular vein–parotid gland–clavicle)
- intercostal, thoracic nodes near the spinal column
- paratracheal nodes along the recurrent laryngeal nerve
- tracheobronchial nodes

These nodes all drain into the right/thoracic lymphatic duct.
- nodes around the celiac trunk (cisterna chili–thoracic duct)

Innervation

- sympathetic nervous system from T4 to T6
- further path of sympathetic innervation: pharyngeal plexus–superior cervical/stellate ganglion–greater splanchnic nerve–celiac plexus
- vagus nerves accompany the esophagus into the abdomen

▓ Anatomy of the Stomach

Location

Division into:
- cardia (stomach entrance)
- fundus (cranial region, filled with air)
- body
- antrum
- pylorus
- greater curvature
- lesser curvature

Table 7.1 Projection onto the wall of the torso.

Structure	Projects to
Greater tuberosity	Fifth ICS on the left
Front of cardia	Left seventh costochondral joint
Back of cardia	T11 on the left costovertebral joint
Lesser curvature	Below the cardia at the level of the seventh costochondral joint on the left parallel to the spinal column up to L1 (T10–L1)
Pylorus	When standing about L3, when lying down L1–L2

ICS, intercostal space.

Cardia and pylorus are relatively fixed points; in between, great variability is possible depending on the state of fullness.

Topographic Relationships

- diaphragm
- indirect: pleura and left lung, pericardium and heart
- ribs 5–8 and costal cartilage 9 on the left
- liver
- celiac trunk and plexus
- omental bursa
- left crus of the diaphragm
- left adrenal gland
- left kidney
- pancreas
- transverse colon
- transverse mesocolon
- left colic flexure
- duodenum (horizontal and ascending part)
- duodenojejunal flexure and start of the jejunum
- spleen

Attachments/Suspensions

- organ pressure
- turgor
- gastrophrenic ligament
- lesser omentum
- greater omentum
- gastrocolic ligament
- gastrolienal ligament
- left phrenicocolic ligament

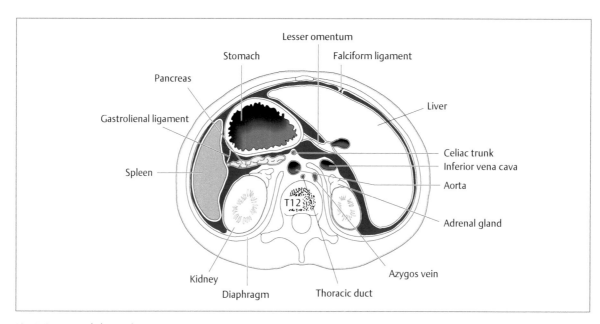

Fig. 7.1 Upper abdominal organs, transverse section.

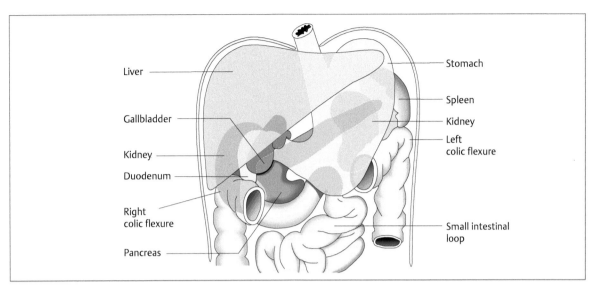

Fig. 7.2 Topographic relationships of the stomach.

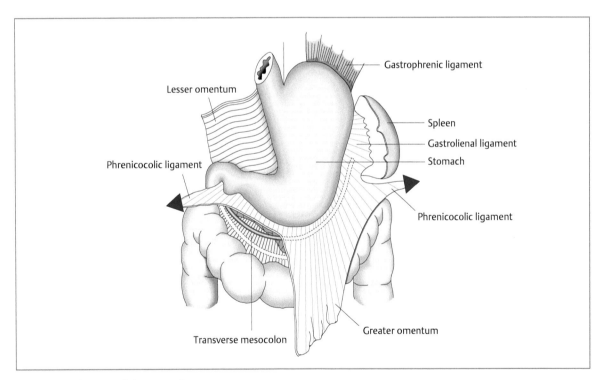

Fig. 7.3 Attachments of the stomach.

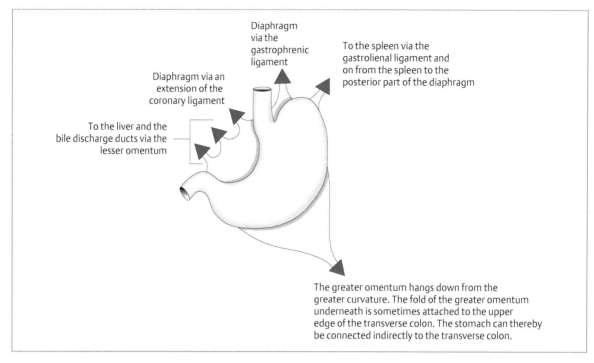

Diaphragm
via the
gastrophrenic
ligament

To the spleen via the
gastrolienal ligament and
on from the spleen to the
posterior part of the diaphragm

Diaphragm via an
extension of the
coronary ligament

To the liver and the
bile discharge ducts via the
lesser omentum

The greater omentum hangs down from the
greater curvature. The fold of the greater omentum
underneath is sometimes attached to the upper
edge of the transverse colon. The stomach can thereby
be connected indirectly to the transverse colon.

Fig. 7.4 Attachments of the stomach, schematic.

Circulation

Arterial

- right gastric artery (from proper hepatic artery)
- left gastric artery (from celiac trunk, anastomosed with the right gastric artery)
- right gastro-omental artery (gastroduodenal artery)
- left gastro-omental artery (splenic artery–celiac trunk)
- gastroduodenal artery (common hepatic artery–celiac trunk)

Venous

Portal vein.

Lymph Drainage

- paracardial lymph nodes
- pancreatic lymph nodes
- splenic nodes
- celiac nodes–thoracic duct (main drainage)

Innervation

- sympathetic nervous system from T6 to T9 via the greater and lesser splanchnic nerves
- further path of sympathetic innervation runs to the celiac and superior mesenteric ganglion
- vagus nerve

Organ Clock

Maximal time: 7–9 a.m.
Minimal time: 7–9 p.m.

Organ–Tooth Interrelationship

For basic information, see page 34.

- Second premolar in the lower jaw on both sides
- Second molar in the upper jaw on both sides

Movement Physiology according to Barral

Mobility

The esophagus has lengthwise mobility. During movements of the head and neck, it must be able to adjust its length.

To transport food, peristaltic waves run through the esophagus during the act of swallowing.

The stomach shows mobility in three planes: frontal, sagittal, and transverse.

Frontal Plane

During inhalation, the diaphragm guides the lateral parts of the fundus of the stomach inferomedially. The distance between the lesser and greater curvature decreases, as does the distance between the fundus and antrum. Looked at from the front, the stomach rotates in a clockwise direction.

The axis of movement is a sagittotransverse axis through the angular incisure of the lesser curvature.

Sagittal Plane

In this plane, the stomach performs a tilt with the cranial parts of the fundus in an anterior direction, accompanied by a simultaneous shift posteriorly in the antral area. The frontotransverse axis of movement runs roughly through the center of the stomach.

Transverse Plane

The stomach performs a rightward rotation along a frontosagittal axis through the inferior part of the esophagus.

Motility

The motions of motility correspond in direction and axis to those of mobility.

Physiology

Proximal and Distal Stomach

The relief structure of the stomach wall serves as a "slide" for the chyme in the direction of the pylorus. The proximal stomach acts as food storage and is marked by continuous tension in the walls.

The distal stomach has the task of mixing, homogenizing, and emulsifying the food. For this purpose, peristaltic waves run from a central pacemaker through the distal stomach. A distension in the stomach stimulates these waves; a distension in the small intestine inhibits the activity of the distal stomach (enterogastric reflex).

The pylorus does not close so tightly that fluids are unable to pass. It relaxes synchronously with each contractile wave of the distal stomach, but only far enough that small food particles can still pass while the large parts are thrown back.

Main Functions of the Stomach

- grinding up solid food, emulsification of fats, predigestion of proteins
- secretion of gastric juice

Gastric Juice

Mucus

Mucus is secreted by the epithelial cells on the surface of the stomach, the side cells of the fundic glands, and the cardiac and pyloric glands.

Bicarbonate

Bicarbonate is secreted by the epithelial cells in the stomach mucosa.

Both components of gastric juice serve to protect the stomach walls from hydrochloric acid (HCl). An H^+ gradient exists across the mucosa, from strongly acid on the lumen side to slightly alkaline on the epithelium side (effect of bicarbonate).

Pepsinogen

Pepsinogen is secreted by the chief cells of the fundic and body glands. At a pH < 3, it is activated into pepsin and cleaves proteins.

Hydrochloric Acid

Hydrochloric acid is secreted by the parietal cells in the fundic glands.

Intrinsic Factor

The intrinsic factor is necessary for the absorption of vitamin B_{12} in the small intestine.

Regulating the Secretion of Gastric Juice

The secretion of gastric juice has several trigger mechanisms.

Cephalic Phase

The secretion of gastric juice is stimulated via the vagus nerve by smell, taste, and glucose deficiency in the brain.

Gastric Phase

Distension of the stomach, amino acids (especially tryptophan and phenylalanine), and Ca^{2+} ions increase the secretion of gastric juice.

Intestinal Phase

This is stimulation by the voiding of chyme into the duodenum. The secretion of gastric juice is inhibited by a strongly acid pH balance in the stomach which inhibits the release of gastrin; this, in turn, inhibits the secretion of HCl in the parietal cells.

Hormones

Gastrin

Gastrin is secreted by the antral glands (two-thirds) and the duodenal mucosa (one-third).

Release Stimulation
- presence of peptides or certain amino acids
- vagal efferents
- high catecholamine concentration in the plasma

Release Inhibition
The pH of gastric juice is < 3.

Functions
- stimulates HCl secretion in the parietal cells
- increases strength and frequency of antral peristalsis
- promotes epithelial growth in the stomach and duodenum
- stimulates the pancreatic acini, bile secretion, and gallbladder contraction

Cholecystokinin

Cholecystokinin (CCK) is secreted in the duodenal and jejunal epithelia.

Release Stimulation
Presence of free fatty acids, peptides, aromatic amino acids, or glucose in the duodenal lumen.

Release Inhibition
Trypsin in the intestinal lumen (protein-cleaving enzyme from the pancreas).

Functions
- stimulates the acinar cells of the pancreas (neutral chloride-rich juice with proenzymes)
- stimulates the secretion of alkaline pancreatic juice rich in bicarbonate
- releases all pancreatic hormones
- promotes pancreatic growth
- stimulates the chief cells of the stomach (⇒ pepsinogen ↑)
- inhibits HCl secretion
- strong stimulator of gallbladder contraction, opens the sphincter of Oddi
- satiety hormone

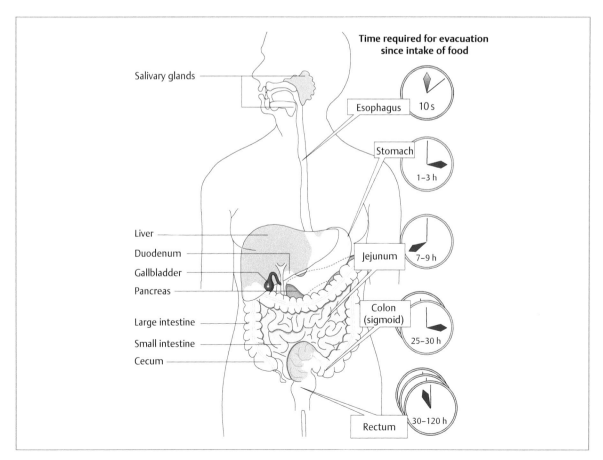

Fig. 7.5 Voiding times from ingestion.

Secretin

Secretin is secreted in the duodenal and jejunal epithelium.

Release Stimulation
Acid chyme.

Functions
- stimulates the secretion of alkaline pancreatic juice rich in bicarbonate
- alkalizes the bile in the bile duct system
- inhibits the resorption of water and salt in the gallbladder
- slows down the emptying of the stomach by inhibiting the stomach muscles
- antitrophic effect on the gastric mucosa

Pathologies

■ Symptoms that Require Medical Clarification

- Tarry stools
- Signs of peritonitis
- Upper abdominal pain that worsens or improves on food intake
- Palpable lymph node at the medial end of the left clavicle (Virchow node)

Hiatus Hernia

Definition

Prolapse of parts of the stomach or of the entire stomach (possibly even of other organs) through the esophageal hiatus into the thorax.

Forms

Sliding Hernia
Movement of the cardia and fundus into the rear mediastinum, with the pointed angle of His being lifted.

Frequently asymptomatic. About 25% of patients develop reflux symptoms; reflux esophagitis is possible (5% of cases).

Paraesophageal Hernia or Rolling Hernia
Protrusion of parts of the fundus into the thorax (past the esophagus and the cardia, which is fixed in its normal location), with a pointed angle of His.

The sphincter continues functioning and reflux is unlikely to occur. Cardinal symptoms are pain in the epigastrium and iron deficiency anemia.

Hybrid forms between the two are possible.

Functional Hernia according to Barral
In cases with similar symptoms, the radiological signs of a hiatus hernia are absent. Such conditions can be caused by a spasm in the gastroesophageal transition or nonphysiologic tissue pulls in the peritoneum, ligaments, or fascia.

Prerequisites for a Healthy Sphincter Function according to Barral

- physiologic pressure conditions in the abdomen and thorax
- causes for pathologic changes: pregnancy, cough, obstipation with impaired defecation
- soft anatomic surroundings that are free from nonphysiologic tissue pulls
- causes for pathologic changes: surgery or effects of inflammation
- physiologic lengthwise tension in the esophagus
- causes for pathologic changes: kyphotic posture or inflammation
- functional diaphragm tension and position
- for healthy sphincter function, the angle of His must be pointed
- normotonic muscle tension at the gastroesophageal transition

Clinical. Roughly 95% of all reflux patients have a hiatus hernia; by contrast, only about 5% of patients with hiatus hernia have reflux disease.

Note
Cardinal symptoms of reflux disease include:
- pain in the epigastrium
- heartburn

Additional symptoms:
- regurgitation
- retrosternal burning
- pain in the middle to lower thoracic spinal column (TSC)

The symptoms are aggravated by:
- lying down
- lifting heavy loads
- bending down
- food intake
- stress
- alcohol
- nicotine

Acute Gastritis

Definition. Acute inflammation of the gastric mucosa with loss of the protective mucus barrier and damage to the mucosa from gastric acid.

Causes
Exogenous factors:
- Bacteria (*Helicobacter pylori*) or toxins (staphylococci)
- alcohol
- medications (acetylsalicylic acid, nonsteroidal anti-rheumatics or NSARs, cytostatics)
Endogenous factors:
- uremia
- portal hypertension
- stress-related ischemia (trauma, burns, shock, competitive sports)
- food allergies

Clinical
- epigastric pain
- nausea
- vomiting
- lack of appetite
- diarrhea
- bad breath

Chronic Gastritis

Definition

Inflammation of the gastric mucosa with infiltration of the lamina propria with immunocompetent cells (lymphocytes, plasma cells, granulocytes).

Causes
- autoimmune disorders
- infection with *H. pylori*
- reflux gastritis

Clinical
Ulcerlike symptoms, e.g.:
- hunger pain
- heartburn
- feeling of fullness
- belching
- flatulence

Gastric Ulcer

Definition. Here, we are dealing with a defect in the walls of the stomach that can also affect the deeper layers of the wall; it is most commonly found in the lesser curvature. Ulcers in the greater curvature raise suspicion of malignancy or are induced by medications.

Causes. Gastric ulcers develop as a result of an imbalance between the production of epithelium-protecting mucus and the secretion of hydrochloric acid. The hydrochloric acid penetrates the mucus barrier and destroys the layers of the stomach walls.
Predisposing factors include:
- infection with *H. pylori*
- chronic gastritis
- increased duodenogastric reflux
- nicotine
- delayed evacuation of the stomach

Clinical
- epigastric pain
- pain aggravated by food intake

Stomach Cancer

Definition. Malignant tumor starting from the epithelial cells of the stomach.

Causes
- People with blood type A have a higher chance of being affected by stomach cancer.
- nitrosamine (metabolic products from bacteria that establish themselves in chronic atrophic gastritis)
- infection with *H. pylori*

Clinical
- nonspecific upper abdominal complaints (feeling of fullness, lack of appetite, nausea, vomiting, hunger pain)
- ulcer symptoms
- weight loss
- distaste for meat
- Virchow node (in about 5 % of cases)
- palpable tumor

Osteopathic Practice

Cardinal Symptoms

- Virchow node
- Pain that occurs a few minutes after eating

Typical Dysfunctions

Adhesions/Fixations and Spasms

These arise after operations, gastritis, gastroenteritis, or blunt stomach trauma.

Ptosis

Favorable factors according to Barral:
- general loss of tonus due to age and the effect of gravity
- asthenic body
- kyphotic posture
- scars
- in women: after pregnancy and childbirth, hormone-related loss of elasticity in the connective tissue
- retroversion of the uterus

Hiatus Hernia

See page 65.

Associated Structural Dysfunctions

- C4–C7
- T1 and first rib on the left
- T6
- T11 and 11th rib posteriorly on the left
- seventh rib anteriorly on the left
- T12–L3
- psoas on the left and iliosacral joint on the left

Atypical Symptoms

A list of symptoms follows that can be explained using osteopathic chains or that result from the patient's history (for an explanation of osteopathic chains, see "Atypical Symptoms" in Chapter 5, page 39):
- humeroscapular periarthritis, more likely on the left
- cervicobrachialgia, more likely on the left
- pain, interscapular or by the superior scapular angle on the left
- large meals between 7 and 9 p.m. trigger the following complaints, which do not occur with large meals outside these times:
  - epigastric pain
  - nausea
  - feeling of fullness and pressure in the right upper abdomen
  - feeling of a lump in the throat
  - increased belching
  - Boas pressure point: hyperparaesthesia paravertebral on the left at the level of T10–T12 in gastric ulcers

In contrast to other authors, Barral additionally lists the following organ-specific symptoms that are signs of gastroptosis:
- constant feeling of heaviness in the abdominal area, which worsens after meals
- working with hands raised above the head or deep inhalations or exhalations cause discomfort in the abdomen
- loosening the belt when eating
- rapid satiation when eating but feeling hungry relatively quickly after eating
- headache that occurs at the end of a larger meal
- flexion in the upper body as protective posture to the distended stomach
- prone position not tolerated for sleeping

Comment. The clinical picture of gastroptosis or a "fish-hook" stomach is very rare in surgery and linked to greater pathologies, e.g., anorexia.

Here it is important to discuss whether the symptoms mentioned by Barral are not rather signs of a functional disorder in the intestines, which responds well to treatment using the described techniques.

Indications for Osteopathic Treatment

- adhesions
- ptosis
- spasms
- hiatus hernia
- humeroscapular periarthritis, more likely on the left
- cervicobrachialgia, more likely on the left
- headache, more likely on the left

Contraindications for Osteopathic Treatment

- fresh scars
- fever
- palpable lymph node at the medial end of the left clavicle (Virchow node)
- If the visceral manipulation triggers strong vegetative reactions, it must be discontinued. These warning signs can include, among others:
  - sweating
  - severe pain with active muscular defense
  - nausea to the point of vomiting

– dizziness
– tendency to collapse
– tachycardia

Notes for Clinical Application

Besides many other causes, stomach diseases and dysfunctions can be traced back to the so-called intestinal tube. This section deals in more detail with this muscular tube, which runs from the stomach cranially through the thorax and finally up to the base of the skull. For this purpose, let us take a closer look at the developmental history of the intestinal tube: in the fourth week of fetal development, the embryo is still stretched out and the future intestinal tube still lies outside the embryo as a yolk sac on the anterior side of the body. Within the next few days, the embryo divides twice, at the end of which the yolk sac is largely integrated into the embryo and the intestinal tube is formed. On the one hand, the embryo folds up from head to tail, so it encloses the yolk sac, pulling it within itself. At the same time, a second folding movement takes place, as if the embryo has covered itself with an overcoat, closing it in front of the abdomen; as a result of this folding in the transverse plane, the yolk sac is incorporated into the embryo. Now the intestinal tube is formed and reaches from the future skull area to the future anus. Nevertheless, the tissues are still undifferentiated at this point, and the intestinal tube hence reaches up to the base of the skull. The differentiation into pharynx, larynx, trachea, and esophagus happens only later. Significant here is the fact that there is a continuous muscular connection from the stomach through the esophagus, larynx, and pharynx up to the base of the skull. As a result, the stomach is ultimately suspended from the base of the skull and hence also affects the sphenobasilar synchondrosis (SBS), which is important for the craniosacral rhythm. Headache that arises in connection with stomach disorders could be explained as a consequence of this.

This tendinous connection of the pharyngeal muscles to the SBS is referred to as the pharyngeal raphe.

The muscular tube from the stomach to the SBS described here is also interesting from another perspective: it is a part of the central tendon, which is a fascial cord that runs through the body from the base of the skull to the pelvic floor, working together as a functional unit. If a dysfunction is present in the body that needs protection, this fascial continuum can help. The ability to carry out a fascial contraction is therefore of great importance: the fascia contracts toward the location of the dysfunction, thereby contributing to its protection. The pharyngo-laryngoesophageal muscle tube operates in this way, and we regard it as part of the central tendon, even though it is not fascia. Nevertheless, the history of its formation and development allows us to place it in close relationship to the deep fascia of the neck and mediastinum.

If the central tendon now participates in a protective

chain in such a way that it results in increased kyphosis of the TSC with protraction of the shoulders (a very common pattern), this posture also has consequences for the stomach:

- The kyphosis goes hand in hand with shortening of the mediastinum.
- The diaphragm is unable to work as effectively because it is forced to work against a higher pressure from the abdominal organs in this posture.
- The esophagus is shortened.

All of these factors result in a change in tonicity in the esophageal hiatus, which forms a key part of the functional seal of the stomach entrance because it also includes the narrowest part of the esophagus. There are two additional bottlenecks: the first is located at the start of the esophagus in the area of the larynx, and the second at the intersection with the trachea and aorta.

To seal the cardia effectively, the following conditions are necessary: a balanced longitudinal tension in the diaphragm and esophagus, a sharp angle of His, a sufficiently small passage of the esophagus through the diaphragm, and good tension in the phrenoesophageal ligament. If just one of these criteria is not met, a real or functional hiatus hernia can result. In the author's opinion, functional hiatus hernias are much more common than generally assumed; their symptoms are, after all, practically identical to those of a real hernia. The treatment of hiatus hernia, whether real or functional, should involve the central tendon from the SBS to the diaphragm.

A functional hiatus hernia can clearly be treated with better results than a real one.

What is Special About the Attachments of the Stomach?
The stomach operates like a mixer: by means of rhythmic peristalsis, it grinds up the food mechanically by repeatedly "flinging" it against the almost completely closed pylorus. Its suspension in the abdominal space is responsible for well-directed peristalsis in the stomach.

Embryologically, the stomach has an anterior and a posterior mesentery, by which it is oriented with the later lesser curvature anteriorly and the greater curvature posteriorly. In the fifth to seventh weeks of embryonic development, the stomach turns by a 90° clockwise rotation into its final position, with the lesser curvature pointing to the right and the greater curvature to the left. The original attachments are preserved but can no longer be as easily recognized as anterior and posterior mesenteries. This is also because other abdominal organs have developed in the mesenteries of the stomach, e.g., the liver and spleen.

The final attachments of the stomach now present as follows: the fundus of the stomach is attached to the diaphragm by means of the gastrophrenic ligament. Subdivided into several ligaments, the former posterior mesentery runs alongside the entire greater curvature. First, the gastrolienal ligament connects the stomach with the spleen. This ligament merges without interruption into the gastrocolic ligament, which connects the stomach with the transverse colon and forms the fixed part of the greater omentum. Including its free part, the greater omentum is the embryological remains of the posterior mesentery. The lesser omentum, which links the stomach to the liver, runs alongside the entire lesser curvature and is the remainder of the former embryological anterior mesentery of the stomach.

When we consider these attachments as a whole, the stomach is suspended like the drum in a washing machine. Mounted and attached securely, but nevertheless capable of great movement, the stomach hangs in the upper abdomen and is able to carry out its peristaltic movements as long as the "mounting" is not thrown off balance. The stomach ligaments must have the proper tension and furthermore pull in the right direction, to serve as an attachment for the stomach, but not become an obstacle as a result of excessive pull. Otherwise the stomach, during peristalsis, has to work against these tensions, which can result in a heightened tonus in the stomach wall and impaired circulation, often leading to gastritis. It appears therefore particularly important to test the stomach ligaments for incorrect tensions and treat accordingly, taking into consideration the fact that the vessels for the stomach run along both the lesser and greater curvatures and that high tension in the ligaments impairs circulation even further.

Osteopathic Tests and Treatment

Mobilization of the Stomach

In the Frontal Plane according to Barral

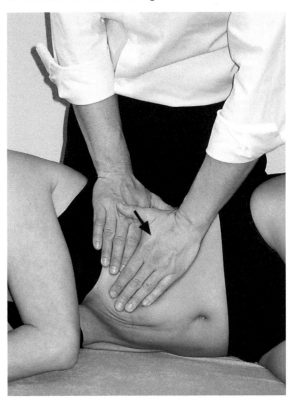

Fig. 7.6

Starting Position
The patient is lying in the side position, facing right. The practitioner stands behind the patient.

Procedure
Place your cranial hand on the lateral costal arch below the diaphragm, approximately at the level of ribs 6–7 on the left.

Place the caudal hand underneath, on top of the ventrolateral lower costal arch.

With both hands, apply pressure medially to press the ribs onto the stomach. Now use both hands simultaneously to mobilize the ribs, and hence indirectly the stomach, in a caudal–medial direction. At the end of the movement, hold the position and carry out a rebound or vibrations.

Proceed similarly to mobilize in the opposite direction in a cranial–lateral direction. Pay particular attention to good contact between the ribs and stomach.

Variation
Place one hand anteriorly and the other posteriorly on the costal arch (pinch grip).

In the Transverse Plane according to Barral

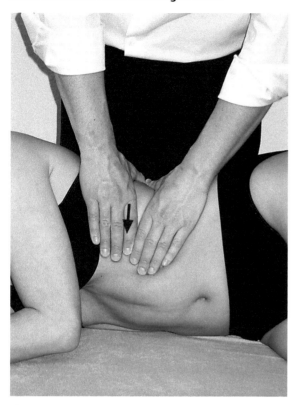

Fig. 7.7

Starting Position
The patient is lying in the side position, facing right. The practitioner stands behind the patient.

Procedure
Place your cranial hand on the lateral costal arch below the diaphragm, approximately at the level of ribs 6–7 on the left. The thumb reaches posteriorly and the fingers anteriorly onto the ribs. In the same way, place the caudal hand underneath, on top of the lateral lower costal arch.

With both hands, apply pressure medially to press the ribs onto the stomach. Now use both hands simultaneously to mobilize the ribs, and hence indirectly the stomach, medially and in a rightward rotation. At the end of the movement, hold the position and carry out a rebound or vibrations.

Proceed similarly to mobilize in the opposite direction laterally and in a leftward rotation. Pay particular attention to good contact between the ribs and stomach.

Variation
Place one hand anteriorly and the other posteriorly on the costal arch (pincer movement).

In the Sagittal Plane according to Barral

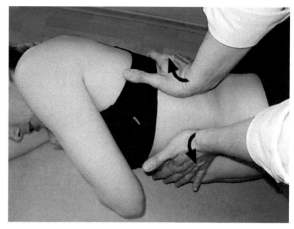

Fig. 7.8

Starting Position
The patient is lying in the side position, facing right. The practitioner stands behind the patient.

Procedure
Place your cranial hand on the lateral costal arch below the diaphragm, approximately at the level of ribs 6–7 on the left. Place the caudal hand on the left costal arch at the level of the seventh to ninth chondrocostal junctions.

With the cranial hand, apply pressure medially, to press the ribs toward the stomach. Now mobilize the stomach via the ribs, with the cranial hand in a cranial–posterior direction and the caudal hand in a caudal–anterior direction. The resulting movement is a wringing out of the stomach.

At the end of the movement, hold the position and carry out a rebound or vibrations.

You can mobilize the opposite direction similarly.

Variation

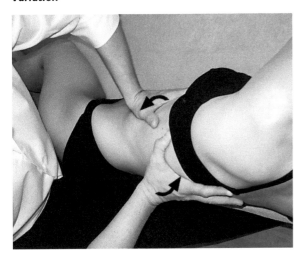

Fig. 7.9

Starting Position
The patient is lying in the side position, facing right, legs bent. The practitioner stands behind the patient.

Procedure
Place the cranial hand on the left costal arch posterior at the level of ribs 6–7 and the caudal hand anterior on the left costal arch with the side of the little finger on the lower edge of the costal arch. In a first step, press the ribs onto the stomach. Now use both hands to mobilize in the sagittal plane by pushing the stomach across the ribs with the cranial hand anterosuperiorly and the caudal hand posteroinferiorly. At the end of the movement, hold the position, initiate vibrations, or mobilize with small rebounds.

Mobilize the opposite direction as well, but with a clearly reduced range of motion.

This variation of the mobilization in the sagittal plane is the mirror image of the technique for mobilization of the liver in the sagittal plane according to Barral (see Chapter 5, page 43).

In the Frontal Plane with Long Arm Lever according to Barral

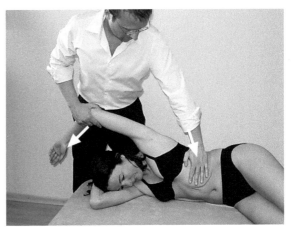

Fig. 7.10

Starting Position
The patient is lying in the side position, facing right. The practitioner stands behind the patient.

Procedure
Place your caudal hand laterally on the lower left costal arch. With the cranial hand, take the patient's left arm and guide it in abduction until you cause the ribs to move as well.

With the caudal hand, apply pressure medially, to press the ribs onto the stomach and mobilize the stomach via the ribs in a caudal–medial direction. The cranial hand fixates the arm in abduction. At the end of the movement, apply a continuous or intermittent pull on the structures. The mobilizing effect pertains to the gliding surface "stomach diaphragm."

Variation
The punctum fixum and punctum mobile can also be switched, so that the caudal hand fixates and the cranial hand mobilizes. Alternatively, both hands can in turn serve as the punctum mobile.

In the Frontal Plane with Long Leg Lever according to Barral

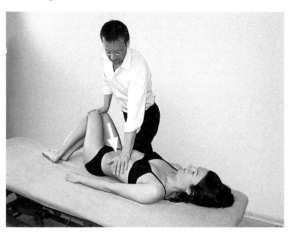

Fig. 7.11

Starting Position
The patient is in the supine position, legs bent. The practitioner stands on the patient's right side.

Procedure
Place your cranial hand with the thenar below the left costal arch onto the stomach. The caudal hand grasps the patient's left knee. With the cranial hand, mobilize the stomach in a cranial–lateral direction; with the caudal hand, pull both knees to the right toward you until the movement reaches the cranial hand. At the end of the movement, apply a continuous or intermittent pull on the structures. Both hands are the punctum mobile.

The mobilizing effect pertains to the gliding surfaces of the stomach with its caudal visceral joints.

Variation
You can also make either hand the punctum fixum and use the other to mobilize.

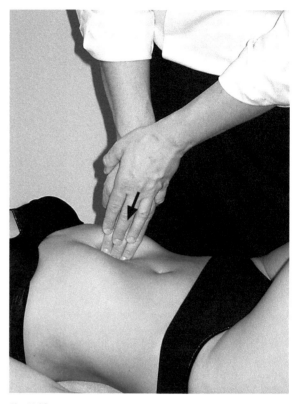

Fig. 7.12

Starting Position
The patient is in the supine position, legs bent. The practitioner stands on the patient's left side.

Procedure
Place the fingers of both hands on the stomach and apply pressure posteriorly until you have made clear contact with the stomach wall. Now oscillate on top of the stomach, i.e., press lightly and intermittently on the stomach with a frequency of 150–180/min. Continue these oscillations for about 2 min.

This technique has a good "de-spasming" effect.

Stretching the Lesser Omentum

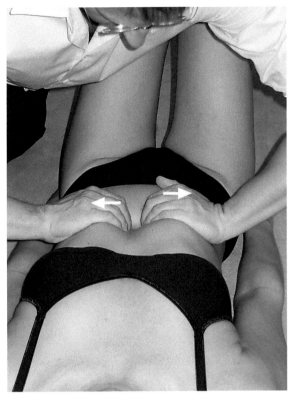

Fig. 7.13

Starting Position
The patient is in the supine position, legs bent. The practitioner stands on the patient's left side.

Procedure
Place the right hand somewhat left of the median line below the xiphoid process with four fingers next to each other on top of the stomach wall. Place the left hand similarly onto the median line next to the right hand.

With both hands, carefully apply pressure posteriorly into the depth of the abdomen. You must proceed slowly, to lower the fascial tensions in this area. This is the only way to reach the lesser omentum.

Once you have penetrated deeply enough with the palpation, gently pull both hands apart laterally, thereby stretching the lesser omentum. Hold the pull of this stretch steady for a maximum of 1 min.

This technique has a reflexive effect on the circulatory structures of the hepatoduodenal ligament.

Pylorus Treatment according to Barral

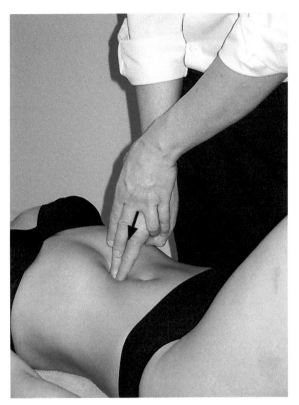

Fig. 7.14

Starting Position
The patient is in the supine position, legs bent. The practitioner stands on the patient's left side.

Procedure
To find the pylorus, look for its approximate projection on the stomach wall. For this purpose, move from the navel about five finger-widths cranially. From there, place your fingers slightly to the right, next to the median line. At this point, slowly slide posteriorly into the abdomen. It is important to proceed slowly, to give the superficial structures time to move out of the way and allow the fascia to relax.

Once you have advanced deeply enough in this palpation, you will usually find a supple, roughly hazelnut-sized solidification within 0.5–1 cm of this palpation point. In most cases, the pylorus is sensitive to palpation.

You can now carry out small circulations, vibrations, or inhibitions on this point, until the tonus and sensitivity are clearly reduced.

Mobilizing the Mediastinum to Improve
Esophageal Mobility according to Barral

Test for Deterioration of Hiatus Hernia
according to Barral

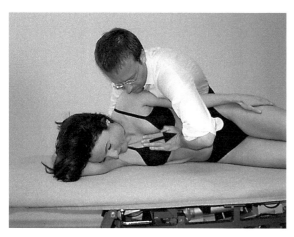

Fig. 7.15

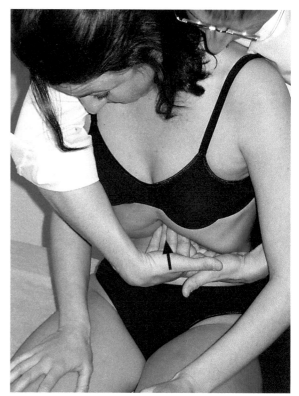

Fig. 7.16

Starting Position
The patient is in the lateral position. The practitioner
stands behind the patient.

Procedure
Place the anterior hand flat on the lower third of the sternum. The posterior hand lies on the spinous processes of
the upper TSC at the level of the manubrium sterni.

With the anterior hand, apply pressure in a caudal–
posterior direction and, with the caudal hand, in a cranial–anterior direction. Release pressure with recoil.
Repeat this procedure 8–10 times.

Then position the hands in such a way that the anterior hand lies on the manubrium and the posterior hand
on the middle TSC at the height of the lower third of the
sternum.

The mobilizing push is now applied anteriorly in a cranial–posterior direction and posteriorly in a caudal–anterior direction.

Starting Position
The patient is sitting. The practitioner stands behind the
patient.

Procedure
Pass your right hand across the patient's right shoulder
on to the abdominal wall, slightly to the left of the
xiphoid process and below the costal arch. Pass the left
hand under the patient's left armpit and place it next to
the right hand.

Bring the patient into a kyphotic position by sliding
both hands simultaneously in a posterior–cranial–right
direction toward the cardia. On arrival there, press the
cardia in the direction of its axis backward–upward–
rightward toward the gastroesophageal junction.

If this pressure triggers typical retrosternal pain in the
patient, possibly with nausea and vegetative reactions,
this is a clear sign of a hiatus hernia and possible reflux
esophagitis.

At the end of the test, abruptly release the pressure. If
this action now causes discomfort in the sense of an
undefined pain, it is most likely that the fascial structures
of the gastroesophageal junction are the cause of the
stomach disorder.

Test for Improvement of Hiatus Hernia according to Barral

Treatment of Hiatus Hernia in the Seated Position according to Barral

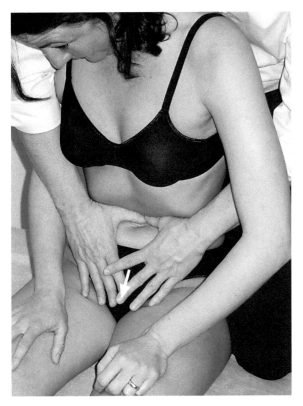

Fig. 7.17

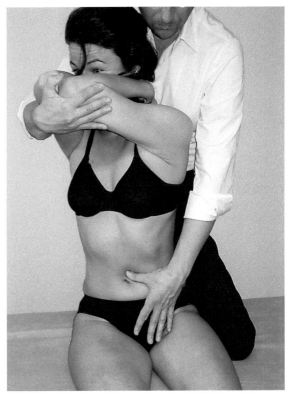

Fig. 7.18

Starting Position

The patient is sitting. The practitioner stands behind the patient.

Procedure

When you carry out the test for deterioration, pressure on the cardia leads to the typical pain. Then palpate along the lesser curvature with both hands caudally, up to the angular incisure. From there, press the stomach slightly caudally and relieve the gastroesophageal junction. The typical symptoms should now be clearly reduced.

This means that a hiatus hernia is likely.

Starting Position

The patient is sitting, hands clasped behind the neck and elbows pointing forward. The practitioner stands behind the patient.

Procedure

Pass both hands below the patient's armpits and place them side by side, slightly to the left of the median line next to the xiphoid process and below the costal arch onto the stomach wall.

Bring the patient into a kyphotic position by sliding both hands simultaneously in a posterior–cranial–right direction toward the cardia. Then palpate along the lesser curvature with both hands caudally, up to the angular incisure.

The left hand remains on this spot and fixes it caudally. The right hand grabs both the patient's elbows and facilitates him or her into an extension-rightward rotation. In this way, the cardia is mobilized caudally. You can hold this mobilization impulse continuously for about 30 sec or apply it intermittently five or six consecutive times.

Treatment of Hiatus Hernia
in the Supine Position

Mobilization of the Gastroesophageal Junction
via the Liver according to Barral

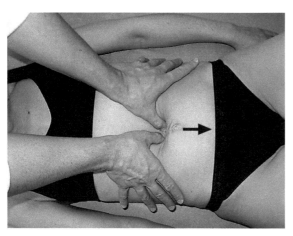

Fig. 7.19

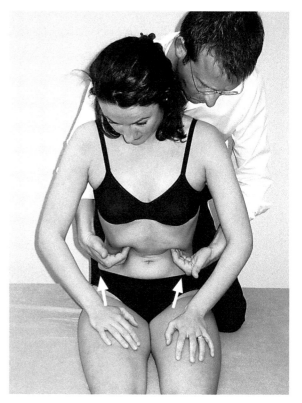

Fig. 7.20

Starting Position
The patient is in the supine position, legs bent. The practitioner stands at the head of the table.

Procedure
Place both hands with the thumbs slightly to the left of the median line and let them sink posteriorly into the stomach until you can palpate the lesser curvature as a sharp edge. Then guide the thumbs along the lesser curvature caudally to the angular incisure. From there, press the stomach caudally with a mobilizing effect on the gastroesophageal junction.

Starting Position
The patient is sitting. The practitioner stands behind the patient.

Procedure
Pass your right hand under the patient's armpit to the right costal arch in the area of the right triangular ligament. Place the left hand similarly under the left costal arch slightly to the side of the medioclavicular line.

Bring the patient into a kyphotic position by sliding your right hand in a posterior–cranial direction and moving the left hand in a posterior–cranial–right direction toward the left triangular ligament.

In the next step, lift the liver with both hands simultaneously cranially and then drop it abruptly. This fall mobilizes the fascial structures of the gastroesophageal junction. Repeat this procedure five or six times.

Treatment of Gastroptosis according to Barral

Starting Position
The patient is sitting. The practitioner stands behind the patient.

Procedure
This procedure aims to give the stomach the greatest possible mobility on its new gliding surface. Do not expect a return to its old position.

Lead your right hand across the patient's right shoulder on to the abdominal wall below the stomach. Pass the left hand under the patient's left armpit and place it next to the right hand.

Now mobilize the stomach with both hands cranially and toward the left shoulder. This mobilization should be performed gently and intermittently, until you notice an improvement in mobility.

Variation
This technique can also be easily performed in the side position, facing to the right. In this case, stand behind the patient and place both hands on the abdominal wall below the stomach. Again, mobilize gently and intermittently in the direction of the left shoulder.

Lastly, the head-down position is also a possible starting position: the advantage here is that the stomach already wants to slide cranially as a result of gravity. The head-down position is also suitable for self-mobilization.

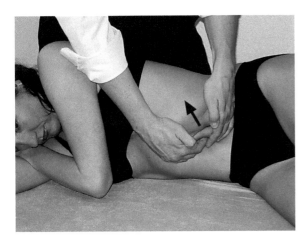

Fig. 7.21

Test and Treatment of Stomach Motility according to Barral

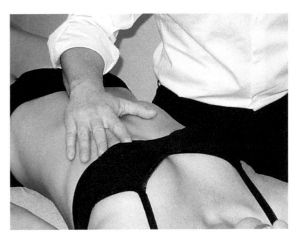

Fig. 7.22

Starting Position
The patient is in the supine position, legs stretched out. The practitioner sits by the patient's right side, facing the head.

Procedure
Lay your right hand without pressure on the patient's abdomen. The thumb lies on the projection of the pylorus, the fingers point in a cranial–lateral direction to the stomach fundus, and the index finger lies on the projection of the lesser curvature. The forearm rests on the abdomen.

Testing Sequence
Detect the motility movement as described above and evaluate the amplitude and direction of the inspiratory and expiratory movements, as well as the rhythm of the movement as a whole. If a disturbance is present in one or both aspects of the motility movement, treat the patient.

Treatment
Motility is treated indirectly by following the unimpaired movement, remaining at the end-point of this movement for several cycles, and then following the impaired movement to the new end-point.

You can also try to increase the range of the free movement (induction), afterward checking whether the limited movement direction has improved.

Repeat this movement again and again until the motility has returned to normal in terms of rhythm, direction, and amplitude.

Fascial Treatment according to Finet and Williame

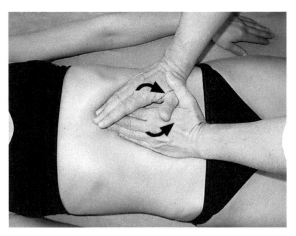

Fig. 7.23

Starting Position
The patient is in the supine position, legs stretched out. The practitioner stands by the patient's left side.

Procedure
Place your right hand with the side of the little finger below the left costal arch, fingers pointing toward the right shoulder. Place the left hand with the side of the little finger to the left of the median line, with the fingertips pointing toward the patient's left shoulder and lying slightly below the right hand.

With both hands, apply the right amount of pressure posteriorly to reach the fascial plane.

Treatment
During inhalation, both hands simultaneously pull caudally. As an additional result, the right hand rotates in a clockwise and the left in a counterclockwise direction. A longitudinal stretch of the stomach results.

During expiration, maintain the position reached. Repeat this procedure until you have reached the end of the fascial movement. In the next exhalation, release the pull.

Repeat the whole treatment four or five times.

Circulatory Techniques according to Kuchera

Arterial Stimulation

- stimulation of the celiac trunk by working on the spinal column
- diaphragm techniques

Venous Stimulation

- liver pump
- stretching the hepatoduodenal ligament
- diaphragm techniques

Lymphatic Stimulation

- lymph drainage on thorax and abdomen
- diaphragm techniques

Vegetative Harmonization

Sympathetic nervous system:
Stimulation of the sympathetic trunk T6–T9 by means of:
- rib raising
- inhibiting the paravertebral muscles
- vibrations
- manipulations
- Maitland technique
- stimulation of the celiac plexus
- diaphragm techniques

Parasympathetic nervous system:
Stimulation of the vagus nerve by means of:
- craniosacral therapy
- laryngeal techniques
- thoracic techniques (recoil)
- diaphragm techniques

Reflex Point Treatment according to Chapman

Location

Esophagus
Anterior. Intercostal space between ribs 2 and 3, near the sternum (on both sides).

Posterior. On T2 halfway between the spinous process and the end of the transverse process, toward the cranial end of the vertebral body (on both sides).

Stomach Secretion (Positive in Stomach Disorders)

Anterior. Intercostal space between ribs 5 and 6, from parasternal to lateral approximately to the level of the mamillary line; present only on the left side!

Posterior. Between the two transverse processes of T5 and T6, halfway between the spinous process and the tip of the transverse process; present only on the left side!

Stomach Tonus

Anterior. Intercostal space between ribs 6 and 7, from parasternal to lateral approximately to the level of the mamillary line; present only on the left side!

Posterior. Between the two transverse processes of T6 and T7, halfway between the spinous process and the tip of the transverse process; present only on the left side!

Pylorus

Anterior. Anterior surface of the sternum, from the manubrium to the xiphoid process.

Posterior. On rib 10, at the level of the costotransverse joint; present only on the right side!

Treatment Principle

Make contact with the reflex point. For this purpose, very gently place a finger on the point and press only lightly. Reflex points are often very sensitive, so it is important to proceed with caution.

The finger remains on the point and treatment is by gentle rotations.

The anterior points are treated first, then the posterior points. Continue with the treatment until you have normalized the sensitivity or consistency of the point.

To conclude, check the anterior points once more. If you fail to notice any change, it is possible that the organ pathology is too great to be influenced quickly via the reflex points, or other dysfunctions are present that must be treated first.

Recommendations for the Patient

- Abstain from eating for about 2–3 hours before treatment.
- Avoid tight pants or belts.
- Avoid working with the hands raised above the head as much as possible.

Patients with Hiatus Hernia

- Consume small meals.
- Do not eat anything in the evening after 6 p.m.
- Place the bed as a whole slightly at an angle, elevating the head.

Patients with Ulcers

- Sugar and industrially processed carbohydrates can promote gastric ulcers.
- Milk consumption causes a short-term rise in the pH level of the stomach, as a result of which there is increased acid production.
- Alcohol and tobacco irritate the stomach.
- Coffee and caffeine-containing drinks can aggravate an ulcer.
- *S*-Methylmethionine and glutamine have a curative effect—raw cabbage juice is rich in these amino acids.
- Strengthen the immune system to fight off helicobacter infections.

8 The Duodenum

Anatomy

General Facts

The duodenum has a total length of 25–30 cm and is shaped like a horseshoe. It extends from T12 to L3, and from the right subcostal to the umbilical area.

It is divided into four parts:
1. Superior part.
2. Descending part.
3. Horizontal part.
4. Ascending part.

The lumen of the duodenum narrows between the superior part and the duodenojejunal flexure from about 4.7 cm to 2.7 cm.

Location

Superior Part

This part is located about 5 cm intraperitoneally. It is the most mobile part of the duodenum. Its location can vary by 4–5 cm, depending on respiration, fullness of the stomach, and posture.

It extends from T12 to L1. The superior part runs from the pylorus cranially, posteriorly, and to the right.

Descending Part

Approximately 10 cm long, this part is located in a secondary retroperitoneal position. It runs vertically toward caudal, more specifically to the right side of the spinal column from L1 to L3(/4).

The excretory ducts of the gallbladder and pancreas enter the descending part posteromedially through the major duodenal papilla (ampulla of Vater). In addition to this common anatomy, there are numerous variations on where these two ducts can enter. An accessory pancreatic duct can enter about 2 cm cranially from the ampulla of Vater, through the minor duodenal papilla (ampulla of Santorini).

Horizontal Part

This part is located approximately 9 cm in a secondary retroperitoneal direction.

Starting from the level of L3(/4), it runs across the vertebral column slightly diagonally upward and leftward to L2.

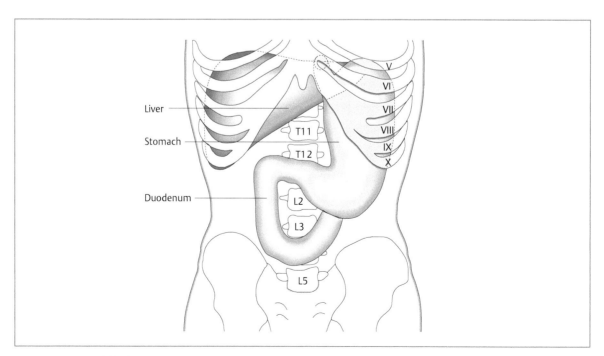

Fig. 8.1 Location of the duodenum.

Ascending Part

This part is located approximately 6 cm in a secondary retroperitoneal direction.

The ascending part rises from L2 to L1 cranially and to the left. It ends with a sharp angle in the duodenojejunal flexure, which again lies intraperitoneally.

Topographic Relationships

Superior Part

- spinal column: in standing position with L2 or L3, in supine position with L1 or L2
- gallbladder
- liver
- inferior vena cava
- head of the pancreas
- hepatoduodenal ligament
- peritoneum

Descending Part

- L1–L3
- transverse colon
- transverse mesocolon
- liver
- ascending colon
- head and excretory ducts of the pancreas
- common bile duct
- ligament of Treitz (suspensory muscle of the duodenum)

- right kidney and renal hilum
- inferior vena cava
- right ureter
- testicular/ovarian vessels
- peritoneum

Horizontal Part

- L2–L3
- root of the mesentery
- superior mesenteric artery and vein
- head of the pancreas
- small intestinal loops
- ligament of Treitz
- psoas major
- aorta
- inferior vena cava
- peritoneum

Ascending Part

- L1 or L2
- minor tuberosity of the stomach and pylorus
- transverse mesocolon
- small intestinal loops
- left psoas major
- ligament of Treitz
- left kidney vessels
- aorta
- left kidney
- peritoneum
- pancreas

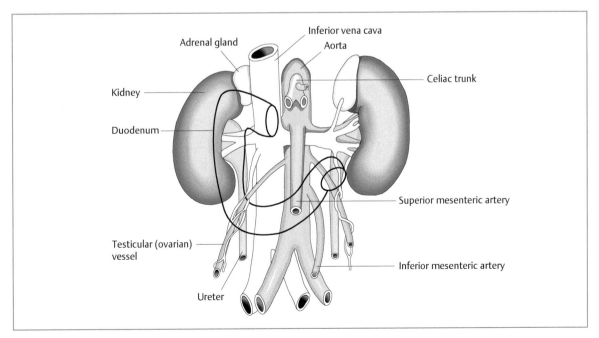

Fig. 8.2 Topographic relationships of the duodenum.

Attachments/Suspensions

- organ pressure
- turgor
- connective tissue in the retroperitoneal space
- hepatoduodenal ligament
- ligament of Treitz

The **ligament of Treitz** (suspensory muscle of the duodenum) consists of smooth and striated muscle fibers. The smooth muscle fibers originate in the superior mesenteric artery and run in a fan-shaped pattern to the ascending part, horizontal part, or duodenojejunal flexure. These fibers radiate into the longitudinal and ring-shaped muscles of the duodenum. The striated muscle fibers originate at the crus of the diaphragm and end at the duodenojejunal flexure.

Circulation

Arterial

- gastroduodenal artery (celiac trunk)
- inferior pancreaticoduodenal artery (superior mesenteric artery)

Venous

- portal vein

Lymph Drainage

Along the vessels to the celiac lymph nodes.

Innervation

Sympathetic nervous system from T9 to T12 via the minor splanchnic nerve to the celiac plexus and the superior mesenteric plexus.

Organ Clock

Maximal time: 1–3 p.m.
Minimal time: 1–3 a.m.

Movement Physiology according to Barral

Mobility

Respiratory movements in the diaphragm, the varying state of fullness in the stomach, and changes in body posture can shift the duodenum as a whole, together with the head of the pancreas caudally by up to one vertebral body, in spite of the fact that it is firmly anchored in the retroperitoneal space. With increasing age, we can also see movement of the duodenum and pancreas caudally. The horizontal part can thereby extend up to the promontory.

According to Barral, the superior part additionally moves toward the ascending part, as a result of which the two arms of the C-shaped duodenum approach each other. The motor of this movement is the diaphragm.

Motility

In the expiratory movement, the superior part moves toward the ascending part, as a result of which the two arms of the C-shaped duodenum approach each other. In the inspiratory phase, this movement is reversed.

Physiology

The structure of the duodenal mucosa corresponds to the basic structure as described in Chapter 12. The circular folds (valves of Kerckring) are particularly pronounced here.

One distinguishing feature of the duodenum is the Brunner glands, which produce large mucus secretions and penetrate the mucosa partly up to the layer of ring-shaped muscle. This mucus secretion contains glycoproteins and bicarbonate to neutralize the acidic chyme.

The cells of the duodenal mucosa have a short lifespan (34–38 hours), which means that we find a fast physiologic renewal of the mucosa. We can interpret this as a defense mechanism against the chyme's acidity, because damaged cells are replaced quickly.

The duodenal mucosa is therefore protected against the acidity of the stomach and the pancreatic enzymes in several ways: by the mucus produced in the Brunner glands, by the bicarbonate in the pancreatic juice, and by rapid renewal of the mucous membranes.

Pathologies

Symptoms that Require Medical Clarification

- Epigastric pain
- Sensitivity to palpation paraumbilically on the right
- Complaints improve significantly on food intake.

Duodenal Ulcer

Definition. Defect in the mucous membrane that can reach into the muscular layer of the mucosa.

Ninety-five percent of ulcers are located in the superior part and in the anterior wall. It occurs three to four times more frequently than a gastric ulcer.

Causes
- Eighty percent of patients are smokers.
- infection with *Helicobacter pylori*
- An excess of acid is present in relation to the protective substances, e.g., bicarbonate.

Clinical
- epigastric pain
- sensitivity to palpation paraumbilically on the right
- significant alleviation of pain on food intake (delayed, night-time, hunger pain)

Osteopathic Practice

Cardinal Symptoms

- Delayed, night-time, hunger pain (epigastric to paraumbilical)
- Pain alleviated by food intake

Typical Dysfunctions

- spasms
- adhesions/fixations
- discharge of bile impaired by papillary spasm or stenosis

Associated Structural Dysfunctions

T12–L1.

Atypical Symptoms

The symptoms can be explained by means of osteopathic chains or results from the patient's history (for an explanation of osteopathic chains, see "Atypical Symptoms" in Chapter 5, page 39).

Pain is in the area of the thoracolumbar junction, sometimes with recurrent structural dysfunctions.

Indications for Osteopathic Treatment

Adhesions/Fixations

Potential causes can be diverse abdominal surgery, as well as inflammatory conditions—also of neighboring organs, e.g., gastric ulcer.

Spasms

Spasms commonly occur together with a duodenal ulcer.

Contraindications for Osteopathic Treatment

- new scars
- acute inflammations, e.g., acute phase of an ulcer or cholecystitis
- a change in symptoms of an ulcer known to the patient, e.g., different quality of pain
- If a treatment of the duodenum triggers obvious vegetative reactions, e.g., severe nausea, vomiting, sweating, dizziness and tendency to collapse, or tachycardia, it must be discontinued.

Osteopathic Tests and Treatment

Treatment of the Sphincter of Oddi (Major Duodenal Papilla) according to Barral

Starting Position
The patient is in the supine position, legs bent. The practitioner stands on the patient's right side.

Procedure
To find the sphincter of Oddi, look for its approximate projection on the stomach wall. For this purpose, move from the navel about three finger-widths cranially. From there, move horizontally in a lateral direction until you cross a line that connects the navel and the right nipple (or the navel and the intersection between the right medioclavicular line and the right costal arch). At this

point, slowly slide posteriorly into the abdomen. It is important here to proceed slowly, so that the superficial intestinal loops or the transverse colon have enough time to move out of the way and the fascia can relax.

Once you have advanced deeply enough in this palpation, you will usually find a supple, roughly pea-sized solidification within 0.5–1 cm of this palpation point. In most cases, the sphincter is sensitive to palpation.

You can now apply small circulations, vibrations, or inhibitions on this point, until the tonus and sensitivity are clearly reduced.

Treatment of the Duodenojejunal Flexure according to Barral

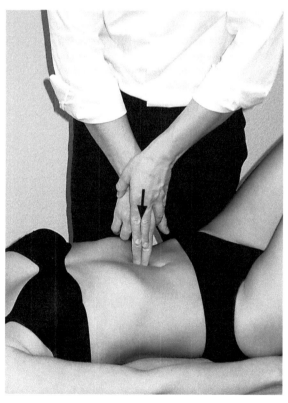

Fig. 8.3

Starting Position
The patient is in the supine position, legs bent. The practitioner stands on the patient's left side.

Procedure
To palpate the duodenojejunal flexure, proceed in a mirror image to the sphincter of Oddi: from the navel, palpate about three finger-widths cranially. From there, move horizontally in a lateral direction until you cross a line that connects the navel and the left nipple (or the navel and the intersection between the left medioclavicular line and the left costal arch). At this point, slowly slide

posteriorly into the abdomen. It is important here to proceed slowly, so that the superficial intestinal loops or the transverse colon have a chance to move out of the way and the fascia can relax.

Once you have advanced deeply enough in this palpation, you will usually find a pressure-sensitive spot within 0.5–1 cm of this palpation point.

You can now apply small circulations, vibrations, or inhibitions on this point, until the tonus and sensitivity are clearly reduced.

The treatment of these two reflex points (sphincter of Oddi and duodenojejunal flexure) causes a reduction in duodenal tonus and in addition general relaxation in the abdomen. These treatments can also be performed independently from duodenal indications as a general visceral treatment.

Mobilization of the Superior Part in the Seated Position via the Liver according to Barral

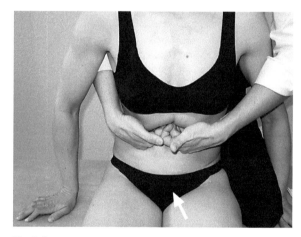

Fig. 8.4

Starting Position
The patient is in the seated position on the edge of the treatment table. The practitioner stands behind the patient.

Procedure
Pass your left arm over the patient's left shoulder onto the right costal arch, medial to the Murphy point. Pass your right arm under the patient's right armpit and place it next to the left hand.

Bring the patient into a kyphotic posture by gliding medially to the gallbladder in a posterior–cranial–lateral direction toward the superior part of the duodenum. Palpate as far as possible in this direction and then make contact with the liver. By lifting the liver cranially, also mobilize the superior part cranially with a pull on the hepatoduodenal ligament. In a second step, "drop" the liver and mobilize the superior part caudally.

De-spasming the Descending and Horizontal Part in Side Position according to Barral

Treating the Angle between the Superior Part and the Descending Part in the Supine Position

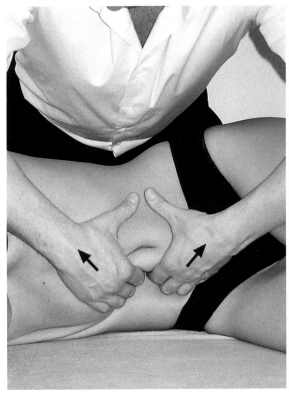

Fig. 8.5

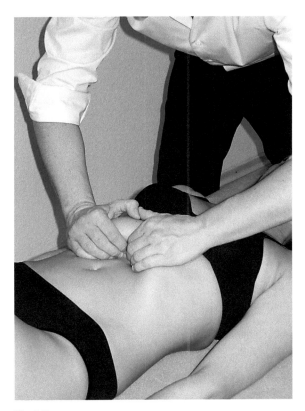

Fig. 8.6

Starting Position
The patient is lying in the side position, facing right, legs slightly bent. The practitioner stands behind the patient.

Procedure
Place both hands on the abdomen medial to the ascending colon and lateral to the loops of the small intestine. The right hand therefore lies below the right costal arch, with the left hand next to it. Now palpate into the depth of the abdomen posteromedially. The loops of the small intestine are in your palms. The fingertips reach the descending part laterally and stretch it simultaneously medially and craniocaudally. This also has an effect on the horizontal part. Hold this position until you notice relaxation in the tissue.

Variation
You can also sit down in front of the patient and proceed in the same way. You merely have to make sure that it is now the left hand that lies below the costal arch.

Starting Position
The patient is in the supine position, legs bent. The practitioner stands at the head of the table by the patient's right shoulder.

Procedure
Place your hands on the abdomen, the left hand slightly lateral to the pylorus projection and the right hand on the medial edge of the projection of the descending part. The fingers of both hands lie next to each other in the direction of the axis of the two parts of the duodenum.

Slide both hands slowly posteriorly into the abdomen in a deep palpation. The tissue lying on top of the duodenum is compressed and fixed onto the superior and descending parts. You have to proceed with caution because otherwise the technique is very painful.

When you have entered deeply enough posteriorly, mobilize the angle in two directions:
1. Facilitate an obtuse angle.
2. Facilitate an acute angle.

Hold the position until you notice a drop in tonicity.

As almost all duodenal ulcers are found in the superior part, you should treat this area in nonacute conditions with particular intensity.

Test and Treatment of Duodenal Motility according to Barral

Fascial Treatment according to Finet and Williame

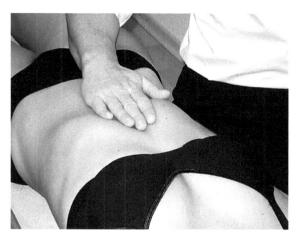

Fig. 8.7

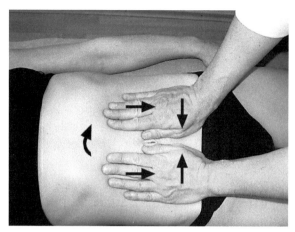

Fig. 8.8

Starting Position

The patient is in the supine position, legs stretched out. The practitioner sits by the patient's right side, facing the head.

Procedure

Place the right hand without pressure on the patient's abdomen. The middle finger lies on the median line, the fingers pointing cranially. The forearm rests on the abdomen.

Testing Sequence

Detect the motility movement: in the expiratory movement, the superior part moves toward the ascending part, as a result of which the two arms of the C-shaped duodenum approach each other. In the inspiratory phase, this movement is reversed.

Evaluate the amplitude and direction of the inspiratory and expiratory movements as well as the rhythm of the movement as a whole.

If a disturbance is present in one or both aspects of the motility movement, treat the patient.

Treatment

Motility is treated indirectly by following the unimpaired movement, remaining at the end-point of this movement for several cycles, and then following the impaired movement to the new end-point.

You can also try to increase the range of the free movement (induction), afterward checking whether the limited movement direction has improved.

Repeat this movement again and again until the motility has returned to normal in terms of rhythm, direction, and amplitude.

Starting Position

The patient is in the supine position, legs stretched out. The practitioner stands by the patient's right side.

Procedure

Place both hands on the abdomen on both sides of the median line. The fingers point cranially, the fingertips lying below the costal arch. With both hands, apply the right amount of pressure posteriorly so that you reach the fascial plane.

Treatment

During inhalation, both hands simultaneously pull caudally and medially, and rotate clockwise. During exhalation, maintain the position reached. Repeat this procedure until you have reached the end of the fascial movement. In the next exhalation, release the pull.

Repeat the whole treatment four or five times.

Circulatory Techniques according to Kuchera

Arterial Stimulation

- stimulation of the celiac trunk and superior mesenteric artery by working on the spinal column
- diaphragm techniques

Venous Stimulation

- liver pump
- stretching the hepatoduodenal ligament
- diaphragm techniques

Lymphatic Stimulation

- lymph drainage on thorax and abdomen
- diaphragm techniques

Vegetative Harmonization

Sympathetic nervous system:
Stimulation of the sympathetic trunk T9–T12 by:
- rib raising
- inhibiting the paravertebral muscles
- vibrations
- manipulations
- Maitland technique
- stimulating the celiac plexus and the superior mesenteric ganglion
- diaphragm techniques

Parasympathetic nervous system:
Stimulation of the vagus nerve by:
- craniosacral therapy
- laryngeal techniques
- thoracic techniques (recoil)
- diaphragm techniques

Recommendations for the Patient

- Avoid nicotine (80% of duodenal ulcer patients are smokers).
- Avoid foods that cause indigestion.

9 The Spleen

Anatomy

General Facts

- Size: 10–12 cm long, 6–7 cm wide, 3–4 cm thick (about fist sized)
- The spleen weighs 150–200 g.
- In its normal size, it is not palpable.

Location

The spleen is located intraperitoneally in the hypochondrium on the left side, at the height of ribs 9–11.

Its longitudinal axis runs approximately by rib 10 from top to bottom, from back to front, and from outside to inside.

The splenic bed is bordered caudally by the phrenicocolic ligament on the left.

Topographic Relationships

- diaphragm
- stomach
- left kidney and adrenal gland
- transverse colon
- phrenicocolic ligament on the left (= sustentaculum lienis)
- pancreas
- ribs 9–11 on the left

Attachments/Suspensions

- organ pressure
- turgor
- phrenicocolic ligament on the left
- gastrosplenic ligament
- splenorenal ligament (previously phrenicolienal ligament)
- pancreaticosplenic ligament

Circulation

Arterial

Splenic artery (via the splenorenal ligament).

Venous

Splenic vein (via the splenorenal ligament).

Lymph Drainage

Pancreaticolienal lymph nodes with connection to celiac, hepatic, and gastric lymph ducts.

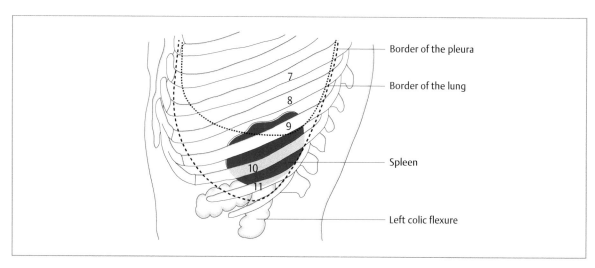

Fig. 9.1 Location of the spleen at the height of ribs 9–11.

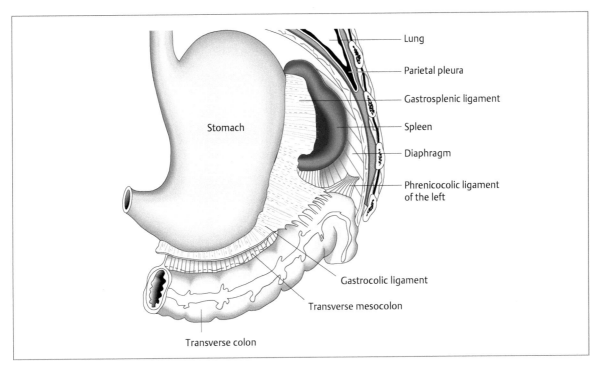

Lung
Parietal pleura
Gastrosplenic ligament
Spleen
Diaphragm
Phrenicocolic ligament of the left

Stomach

Gastrocolic ligament
Transverse mesocolon
Transverse colon

Fig. 9.2 Attachments of the spleen.

Innervation

- sympathetic nervous system from T5 to T9 via the major splanchnic nerve and switching in the celiac plexus
- vagus nerve

Organ Clock

Maximal time: 9–11 a.m.
Minimal time: 9–11 p.m.

Organ–Tooth Interrelationship

For basic information, see page 34.

- First back tooth in the lower jaw on the left
- First molar in the upper jaw on the left

Movement Physiology according to Barral

Mobility

The spleen follows the movements of the diaphragm: during inhalation, we see a shift in a caudal–medial direction; during exhalation it is in the opposite direction.

The spleen's position is also affected by shifts in body posture and changes in the tension and length of the phrenicocolic ligament on the left and the transverse colon. A full stomach similarly displaces the spleen anteroinferiorly.

Physiology

- removal of old or damaged blood cells (especially erythrocytes), thrombocytes, microorganisms, or immune complexes
- antigen-induced differentiation and proliferation of B and T lymphocytes
- storage of thrombocytes and erythrocytes

Pathologies

Symptoms that Require Medical Clarification

- Splenomegaly

Splenomegaly

Definition. This term refers to an enlarged spleen. The increase in size can be so great that the spleen becomes palpable.

Causes. Splenomegaly is a possible symptom in different pathologies, such as:
- blood and lymph diseases (lymphoma, leukemia, hemolytic anemia)
- liver diseases (cirrhosis, hepatitis)
- rheumatic disorders

- portal hypertension
- storage disorders (e.g., amyloidosis)
- infectious diseases (e.g., malaria, typhoid)
- sarcoma
- abscess
- echinococcal cyst

Clinical. The spleen is palpable or diagnosable by technical means because it is enlarged.

In cases where the enlargement of the spleen is gradual, symptoms arise as a result of the displacement. In cases with a more rapid enlargement, we can see coliclike pain in the left upper abdomen radiating into the left shoulder.

As splenomegaly is often a secondary symptom, we must pay attention to other signs of disease.

Hypersplenism

Definition. The occurrence of anemia, granulocytopenia, or thrombocytopenia as the result of splenic hyperfunction. This hyperfunction frequently occurs together with a splenomegaly.

Causes. See page 89 (splenomegaly).

Clinical. See page 89 (splenomegaly).
Changes in the blood count.

Osteopathic Practice

Cardinal Symptom

- Splenomegaly

Typical Dysfunctions

A typical dysfunction in the sense of an adhesion/fixation, ptosis, or spasm does not exist in the spleen.

Associated Structural Dysfunctions

Ribs 9 and 10 on the left.

Atypical Symptoms

A list of symptoms follows that can be explained by means of osteopathic chains or result from the patient's history (for an explanation of osteopathic chains, see "Atypical Symptoms" in Chapter 5, page 39):
- stitches in the left side
- weak immune system

Indications for Osteopathic Treatment

Treatment of the spleen is recommended for the purpose of stimulating the immune system.

Contraindications for Osteopathic Treatment

- splenomegaly
- hypersplenism

Notes for Clinical Application

In addition to the liver, small intestine, and thymus, the spleen is one of the immunocompetent organs. Immunocompetent organs are organs that take on a function in our immune system, even if only temporarily (e.g., the thymus).

The immune system can be impaired in two ways: we can see a weakening of the immune system. Such patients have frequent infections of the respiratory tracts. Inflammation of the sinuses, larynx, bronchial tubes, or the lung is common in such cases. This type of immune disorder can already affect infants. Even children who are still protected by their mother's immunity (breastfed) can also experience abnormally frequent critical respiratory tract infections as a sign of a weakened immune defense.

Another sign of a weakened immune system is frequent infections of the urogenital tract. In particular, when we see recurrent bladder inflammations in patients who have never had, or not had for a very long time, such infections, a close look at the liver, small intestine, spleen, and, when still active, thymus, is worthwhile.

In addition, however, the immune system can be disturbed in the sense of an overreaction. The results are then allergies to pollen, animal hair, foods, etc. The exaggerated response can be even greater, as a result of which we see neurodermatitis, bronchial asthma, or autoimmune disorders.

In all cases where these allergic disorders become stronger or weaker during different stages of life, i.e., where we see a "movement" in these allergies, and the allergy-triggering substances do not affect the patient excessively, treatment with osteopathy is indicated. It is not uncommon to find dysfunctions in the liver, small intestine, spleen, or thymus, which disturb the body's immune defense. We should take a close look at these organs in cases of both generalized weakness and hypersensitivity of the immune defense system.

In addition, it is important to diagnose and, if necessary, treat the diseased organs themselves. The lungs and the bladder, in particular, are organs that by their nature come into frequent contact with pathogenic organisms, and therefore possess a well-developed defense system of their own.

If this defense is weakened or hypersensitized, we should strengthen the immunocompetence of the organs using structural or circulatory treatments.

Lastly, let us deal with one particular stress situation of the immune system in more detail. We all have phases of life that are particularly stressful—stages in life that are taken up by strong negative factors, i.e., stress is experienced as a burden rather than a motivation. Such states can be caused by either exceptional situations at work or private stress situations such as separation or illness. Unfortunately, this stress also affects children: they suffer most from separation of parents, even if this is not always apparent. Immense pressure at school can also weigh heavily on them, a pressure that unfortunately often stems from the parents.

To manage stress, our body utilizes the hormone cortisol, which is produced in the adrenal glands. It functions well as long as the stressful situation does not persist for too long. When this phase becomes a permanent state, however, the high level of cortisol has an immunosuppressive effect on the body. In such cases, we see frequent and recurrent infections. The respiratory and urogenital tracts are again affected most frequently, but less common viral disorders such as herpes zoster can also occur.

If the disturbance of the immune system is massive, first we have to identify and eliminate the triggering stress factor, before we have a chance to regenerate the body's defense.

Osteopathic Tests and Treatment

Test and Stretch of the Phrenicocolic Ligament

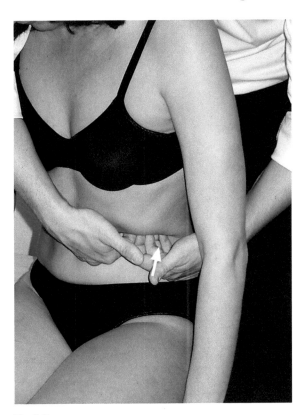

Fig. 9.3

Starting Position
The patient is sitting. The practitioner stands behind the patient.

Procedure
Place the fingertips of both hands on the abdomen below the left costal arch. Palpate the transverse colon and follow it in a left lateral direction to the left colic flexure. Slightly lateral to the flexure, you can palpate the ligament running left to the diaphragm.

Lateral flexion to the left relaxes the phrenicocolic ligament; contralateral lateral flexion tightens it.

Testing Sequence
Evaluate the tightness and sensitivity of the ligament in both the tightened and the relaxed state.

Treatment
Press the ligament in a cranial–lateral direction to stretch it. At the same time, a contralateral lateral flexion can increase the stretch.

Stretch of the Gastrosplenic Ligament

Spleen Pump

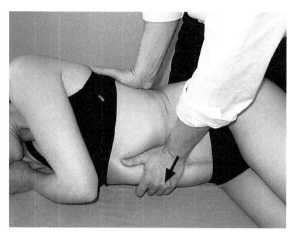

Fig. 9.4

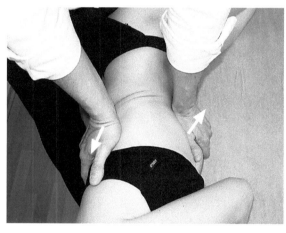

Fig. 9.5

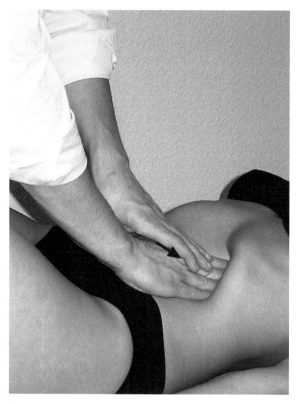

Fig. 9.6

Starting Position

The patient lies in the side position, facing right. The practitioner stands behind the patient.

Procedure

Place your cranial hand on top of rib 10, on the right above the spleen. With the caudal hand, find the greater curvature of the stomach and palpate it with the thenar.

With the caudal hand, mobilize the stomach medially, while at the same time using the cranial hand to fixate rib 10 on the spleen and mobilize both posteriorly and slightly cranially.

This action stretches the ligament. Hold the position reached for up to 30 sec. You can repeat this technique several times.

Starting Position

The patient is in the supine position, legs bent. The practitioner stands on the patient's right side.

Procedure

Place the fingers of your right hand with the side of the little finger below the left costal arch. Place the left hand on top of the right hand. With both hands, oscillate in the direction of the spleen, i.e., press lightly and intermittently in a cranial–lateral direction with a frequency of 150–180/min. Continue these oscillations for about 2 min.

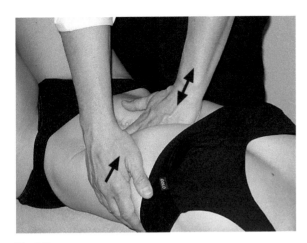

Fig. 9.7

Variation

Place the left hand with the side of the little finger below the left costal arch. Place the right hand on top of the lateral costal arch, on the left side above the spleen (guiding structure is rib 10).

The right hand pulls the costal arch slightly in a caudal–medial direction toward the left hand. The left hand stimulates the spleen by light rhythmic oscillations toward the right hand.

Fascial Treatment according to Finet and Williame

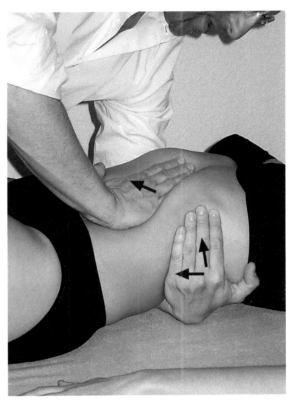

Fig. 9.8

Starting Position

The patient is in the supine position, legs stretched out. The practitioner stands on the patient's right side.

Procedure

Pass your left hand under the patient and place it below the left costal arch posterolateral at the height of the spleen. Place the right hand with the side of the little finger below the left costal arch, with the fingertips pointing toward the right armpit. With both hands, apply enough pressure (with the right hand posteriorly and the left hand medially) to reach the fascial plane.

Treatment

During inhalation, pull with both hands caudally. The right hand also pulls medially and the left moves toward the median line.

During exhalation, maintain the position reached. Repeat this procedure until you have reached the end of the fascial movement. In the next exhalation, release the pull.

Repeat the whole treatment four or five times.

Circulatory Techniques according to Kuchera

Arterial Stimulation

- stimulation of the celiac trunk by working on the spinal column
- diaphragm techniques

Venous Stimulation

- liver pump
- stretching the hepatoduodenal ligament
- diaphragm techniques

Lymphatic Stimulation

- lymph drainage on thorax and abdomen
- diaphragm techniques

Vegetative Harmonization

Sympathetic nervous system:
Stimulation of the sympathetic trunk T5–T9 by:
- rib raising
- inhibiting the paravertebral muscles
- vibrations
- manipulations
- Maitland technique
- stimulation of the celiac plexus
- diaphragm techniques

Parasympathetic nervous system:
Stimulation of the vagus nerve by:
- craniosacral therapy
- laryngeal techniques
- thoracic techniques (recoil)
- diaphragm techniques

Reflex Point Treatment according to Chapman

Location

Anterior. Intercostal space between ribs 7 and 8 on the left side, near the rib cartilage.

Posterior.
Between the two transverse processes of T7 and T8, halfway between the spinous process and the tip of the transverse process; present only on the left side!

Treatment Principle

Make contact with the reflex point. For this purpose, very gently place a finger on the point and press only lightly. Reflex points are often very sensitive, so it is very important to proceed with caution.

The finger remains on the point and treatment is by gentle rotations.

The anterior points are treated first, then the posterior points. Continue with the treatment until you have normalized the sensitivity or consistency of the point.

To conclude, check the anterior points once more. If you fail to notice any change, it is possible that the organ pathology is too great to be influenced quickly via the reflex points, or other dysfunctions are present that must be treated first.

Recommendations for the Patient

- To support the immune system through the diet, reduce the consumption of industrially processed carbohydrates, saturated fats, and alcohol as much as possible.
- The following foods strengthen the immune system:
  - lean meat
  - low-fat dairy products
  - whole grains
  - fresh fruit and vegetables
  - fish
  - nuts
- The listed foods contain micronutrients that strengthen the body's immune defense. These micronutrients include:
  - vitamin A
  - vitamin B_6
  - vitamin C
  - vitamin E
  - selenium
  - zinc

10 The Pancreas

Anatomy

General Facts

The pancreas is 14–18 cm long and weighs 70–80 g. It is a gland with exocrine and endocrine features.

Division

- head of pancreas with the uncinate process
- body of pancreas
- tail of pancreas
- pancreatic duct (Wirsung)
- accessory pancreatic duct (Santorini)

Location

The pancreas is a secondarily retroperitoneal organ. It lies on the median line roughly at the level L1–L2, with the head lower than the tail: the axis of the body is inclined toward the upper left approximately 30° to the horizontal line.

The accessory pancreatic duct, if present, enters the duodenum 2–3 cm above the major duodenal papilla.

Topographic Relationships

- duodenum
- L2–L3 (head of pancreas), covered by the right crus of the diaphragm
- common bile duct
- aorta
- inferior vena cava
- left renal vein

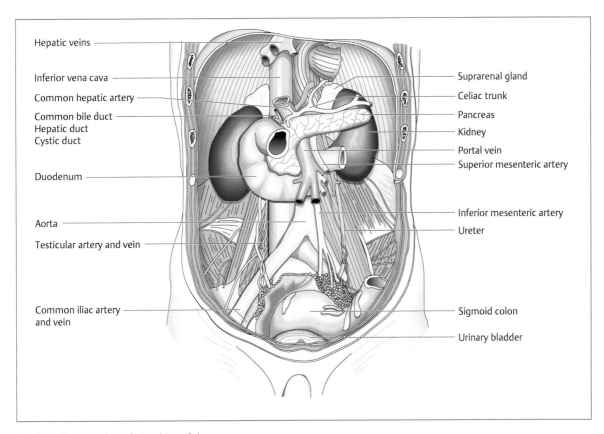

Fig. 10.1 Topographic relationships of the pancreas.

- pylorus
- superior mesenteric artery and vein
- duodenojejunal flexure
- omental bursa
- stomach
- kidneys
- transverse mesocolon (divides the pancreas into a sub- and a supramesocolic part)
- transverse colon
- left colic flexure
- splenic vein
- peritoneum
- spleen
- lesser omentum
- portal vein

Attachments/Suspensions

- organ pressure
- turgor
- attachments of connective tissue in the retroperitoneal space
- pancreaticosplenic ligament
- retropancreatic fascia (Treitz)
- transverse mesocolon
- duodenum

Circulation

Arterial

- superior mesenteric artery
- gastroduodenal artery (from the common hepatic artery)
- splenic artery

Venous

- superior mesenteric vein
- portal vein (from the splenic vein and pancreaticoduodenal veins)

Lymph Drainage

- direct lymphatic connections to nearby organs (duodenum)
- via celiac lymph nodes to the gastric and hepatic lymph nodes on the left side of the body
- mediastinal and cervical lymph nodes
- pancreaticolienal lymph node and pylorus
- mesenteric and periaortal lymph nodes

Innervation

- sympathetic nervous system from T5 to T9 (sometimes also T10 and T11) via the major splanchnic nerve, with switching in the celiac plexus
- vagus nerve

Organ Clock

Maximal time: 9–11 a.m.
Minimal time: 9–11 p.m.

Organ–Tooth Interrelationship

For basic information, see page 34.

- First back tooth in the lower jaw, right side
- First molar in the upper jaw on the right side

Movement Physiology according to Barral

Mobility

Due to the good fascial anchoring in the retroperitoneal space, it is impossible to detect a separate mobility. Nevertheless, the movements of the neighboring organs and the diaphragm cause pushing and pulling on the pancreas.

Motility

With a hand that rests on the projection of the pancreas on the abdomen (fingers pointing to the tail, thenar lies above the head), we can detect a wave from the heel of the hand to the fingertips during exhalation. During inhalation, the wave runs in the opposite direction.

Physiology

The pancreas is a gland with exocrine and endocrine features. The endocrine parts, the islets of Langerhans, are distributed throughout the entire pancreas with accumulations in the body and tail. The cells in the islets of Langerhans produce the hormones that are responsible for regulating blood sugar: insulin, glucagon, and somatostatin.

Insulin

Insulin is synthesized in the β cells of the islets of Langerhans (approximately 2 mg/day) and lowers the blood sugar level by making the cell wall of each body cell permeable to glucose. In addition, insulin assists in the uptake of different amino acids into the cell.

In the liver, it initiates a variety of metabolic processes:

- glycogen synthesis and inhibition of glycogenolysis
- synthesis of lipids and inhibition of lipolysis
- inhibition of protein breakdown

Glucagon

Glucagon is produced in the α cells of the islets. It is the "insulin antagonist": by promoting glycogenolysis and gluconeogenesis in the liver, it raises the blood sugar level.

Somatostatin

The δ cells synthesize this hormone. It suppresses the release of insulin and glucagons, and decreases digestive activity by reducing intestinal peristalsis and inhibiting the secretion of digestive juices. Its function is to maintain the glucose level as much as possible.

The **exocrine gland part** of the pancreas secretes juice into the pancreatic duct. As a result of its activity, approximately 1–1.5 L of "abdominal saliva" thus reaches the duodenum per day.

This secretion consists of:

- bicarbonate to neutralize the acidic chyme from the stomach
- trypsinogen and chymotrypsinogen (enzymes for digesting protein)
- α-amylase (also present in the saliva of the mouth) for cleaving carbohydrates
- lipase (enzyme for cleaving fat)

The enzymes of this "abdominal saliva" are not yet activated in the pancreas. It is only after contact with bile or the enterokinase in the duodenal juice that they are activated and begin working. If this activation takes place in the pancreas, it results in autodigestion and the symptoms of acute pancreatitis.

Pathologies

Symptoms that Require Medical Clarification

- Icterus
- Pain in the depth of the upper abdomen with back pain in the area of the lower thoracic spinal column, radiating beltlike from the back to the front
- "Rubber stomach"

Acute Pancreatitis

Definition. Inflammation of the pancreas with disturbance of exocrine and endocrine functions.

Causes
- biliary tract disorders (40–50%)
- alcohol abuse (30–40%)
- idiopathic (10–30%)

Rare causes include:
- medications (diuretics, β blockers, glucocorticoids, antibiotics, nonsteroidal antirheumatics)
- trauma
- infections (mumps, Coxsackievirus)
- hypercalcemia (e.g., hyperparathyroidism)
- hyperlipoproteinemia
- papillary stenosis

Clinical
- guiding symptom: severe upper abdominal pain, arising approximately 8–12 hours after a large meal or alcohol abuse, with pain radiating into the back and ringlike to the left around the torso
- shock

Chronic Pancreatitis

Definition. Chronic inflammation of the pancreas is characterized by persistent or recurrent pain with usually irreversible morphologic changes in the pancreatic parenchyma and functional disturbances in the pancreas.

Causes
- alcohol (70–90%)
- idiopathic (10–25%)

Rare causes include:
- anomalies in the pancreatic duct system
- hyperparathyroidism
- trauma
- abuse of analgesics

Clinical
- upper abdominal pain
- nausea, vomiting
- icterus
- depression
- diabetes mellitus
- constipation
- thrombophlebitis
- excretory insufficiency
- weight loss
- steatorrhea
- diarrhea
- meteorism
- edemas

When approximately 90% of pancreatic tissue is destroyed, we see steatorrhea as a sign of maldigestion, as well as symptoms of fat-soluble vitamin deficiency (night blindness, clotting disorders, osteomalacia).

Pancreatic Cancer

Definition.   Malignant tumor of the pancreas, usually originating in the epithelium of the duct system.

Causes.   Unknown genesis. Under discussion are alcohol, nicotine, and coffee consumption as predisposing factors.

Clinical.   No early symptoms.
- weight loss
- recurrent thrombophlebitis
- back pain
- obstructive icterus

Osteopathic Practice

Cardinal Symptoms

> - Pain in the thoracolumbar junction and belt shaped above the navel
> - "Rubber stomach"

Typical Dysfunctions

Disturbed endocrine or exocrine gland function.

Associated Structural Dysfunctions

- T9
- iliosacral joint on the left
- irritation of the levator scapulae attachment on the left

Atypical Symptoms

A list of symptoms follows that can be explained by means of osteopathic chains or result from the patient's history (for an explanation of osteopathic chains, see "Atypical Symptoms" in Chapter 5, page 39):
- epigastric complaints after eating (nausea, feeling of fullness, feeling of pressure)
- fatigue
- slightly forward-bent protective posture
- discolored stools

In contrast to other authors, Barral also lists the following organ-specific symptoms:
- hot flashes after eating
- pain via the median scapular angle on the left (especially after large/heavy meals)
- flat breathing at the conclusion of meals and the start of the digestive phase
- sensitivity to smells, especially heavy perfumes
- preference for heavily spiced or sour foods

Indications for Osteopathic Treatment

The indications are based on the atypical symptoms and associated structural dysfunctions.

Contraindications for Osteopathic Treatment

- acute pancreatitis
- icterus
- tumors
- infections
- fever

If a treatment of the pancreas triggers obvious vegetative reactions, e.g., severe nausea, vomiting, sweating, dizziness, tachycardia, and tendency to collapse, it must be discontinued.

The pancreas must be considered in the functional context of the liver and gallbladder. Disease in one of these organs can lead to pathology in the others:

A gallstone that occludes the papilla of Vater can, when bile backs up into the pancreas, cause acute pancreatitis. In the reverse direction, the swelling of the pancreas in acute pancreatitis can constrict the common bile duct, resulting in posthepatic icterus.

Notes for Clinical Application

In osteopathy, the pancreas cannot be looked at in isolation because it has a functional connection to the liver, gallbladder, and duodenum. To illustrate this point, let us digress into the anatomy here.

The common bile duct is formed from a union of the hepatic duct with the cystic duct on the posterior side of the liver. Together with the portal vein and proper hepatic artery, it runs in the hepatoduodenal ligament caudally. This part of the bile duct hence lies intraperitoneally. The ligament ends at the upper edge of the first part of the duodenum. The bile duct now continues on behind the superior part of the duodenum caudally. From here on, it maintains this retroperitoneal position until it leads into the descending part of the duodenum. On the way to the major duodenal papilla, it passes through the head of the pancreas, reaches the area where it ends on the posterior side of the descending part of the duodenum, and runs diagonally through the intestinal wall. In this way, the smooth muscle fibers of the intestinal wall surround the bile duct as sphincter muscles and together with it form the major duodenal papillae (papilla of Vater, sphincter of Oddi). The pancreatic duct also joins here, in such a way that it delivers its secretion near the papilla into the bile duct.

In its initial section, the common bile duct is about twice as large in diameter as in the area by the papilla. This is highly significant because a gallstone that can still easily fit through the cranial part of the duct can get stuck in its final section. This situation has two results: first, it leads to a retrograde backflow of bile into the liver, which can cause an icterus; second, the bile backs up into the excretory duct of the pancreas, which can trigger acute pancreatitis. These are two examples of the way in which a disease of one organ in this functional series of upper abdominal organs can lead to a disease or symptom in another organ. Let us give a few more examples.

The superior part of the duodenum is the location that is most frequently affected by ulcers in the duodenum. Such a disorder can cause hypertonicity in the muscles of the duodenal wall, which we refer to in osteopathic terms as a spasm of the organ. A spasmic superior part exerts a higher than normal pressure on its environment. Most affected by this is the common bile duct behind the beginning of the duodenum because it is unable to avoid this pressure in the retroperitoneal space. Even a discrete constriction of the lumen of the bile discharge duct results in backflow of bile into the liver, with posthepatic icterus in extreme cases.

Such a spasm can also reach into the descending part of the duodenum and there affect the papilla as well. A papilla spasm also causes a backflow of bile into the liver. Another reason for a papillary spasm is psychosomatic stress, which can have far-reaching effects, to the point of causing signs typical of a stone disorder in the gallbladder with intolerance of fat, coffee, etc., but no verifiable evidence of gallbladder inflammation or stones. A papillary spasm is characterized by pronounced sensitivity to pressure.

A disorder of the pancreas also has an effect on the common bile duct: a swelling in the head section of the pancreas, as we found in acute or chronic pancreatitis or in cancer of the pancreatic head, can constrict the bile duct and cause the already mentioned backflow of bile into the liver.

Thus there are several good reasons why the liver, gallbladder, duodenum, and pancreas form a functional unit. The question is: how can the osteopath accommodate this fact? Certainly the most likely organ in this group to show dysfunctions is the liver (see also Chapter 5, page 39). Knowing that disorders in the other three organs can have a detrimental effect on the liver, osteopathic diagnosis and, if indicated, therapy should also extend to these organs.

For the treatment of the pancreas itself, only a few techniques are available. As a result of this, it is all the more important to look at its surroundings: first to mention here are the duodenum and stomach. If you promote healthy mobility in these organs, you have also done a lot for the pancreas—as, in particular for the pancreas, the circulatory techniques according to Kuchera offer excellent treatment opportunities.

Finally, let us also discuss briefly a very common dysfunction of the pancreas, namely relative exocrine pancreatic insufficiency. This term refers to a temporary lack of enzymes in the pancreatic juice and resulting digestive problems, which manifest in occasional diarrhea and food intolerances. This disorder is best characterized as follows: these are patients who appear to be affected by every gastrointestinal disorder. Falling ill with diarrhea 10–12 times a year is not uncommon. Sometimes the patient tolerates fatty foods, sometimes not. The patient's own explanations might state that he or she has yet again caught a virus or that last night's food must have been bad.

This excretory insufficiency of the pancreas responds well to treatment with osteopathy, especially with circulatory techniques.

Osteopathic Tests and Treatment

Fascial Stretch of the Pancreas in Longitudinal Axis according to Barral

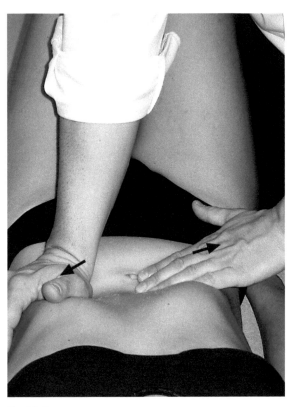

Fig. 10.2

Test and Treatment of Pancreatic Motility according to Barral

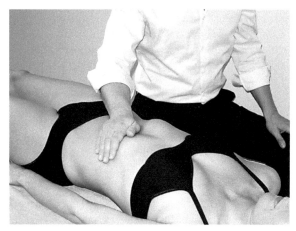

Fig. 10.3

Starting Position
The patient is in the supine position, legs stretched out. The practitioner sits by the patient's right side.

Procedure
The right hand of the practitioner rests without pressure on the projection of the pancreas on the abdomen—the thenar on the head, the fingertips on the tail. The forearm also rests on the abdomen.

During exhalation, you will notice a wavelike movement from the heel of the hand to the fingertips, during inhalation it is in the opposite direction.

Testing Sequence
Detect the motility motion and evaluate the amplitude and direction of the inspiratory and expiratory movements as well as the rhythm of the movement as a whole. If a disturbance is present in one or both aspects of the motility movement, treat the patient.

Treatment
Motility is treated indirectly by following the unimpaired movement, remaining at the end-point of this movement for several cycles, and then following the impaired movement to the new end-point.

You can also try to increase the range of the free movement (induction), afterward checking whether the limited movement direction has improved.

Repeat this movement again and again until the motility has returned to normal in terms of rhythm, direction, and amplitude.

Starting Position
The patient is in the supine position, legs bent. The practitioner stands on the patient's right side at the height of the pelvis.

Procedure
Place your left hand on the abdomen, with the fingers on the projection of the head of the pancreas. The right hand is placed with the thenar on the projection of the tail of the pancreas. Now apply gentle pressure posteriorly with both hands, compressing the superficial tissue on top of the pancreas. When you have reached the fascial plane of the pancreas, stretch with both hands simultaneously along the longitudinal axis of the pancreas and hold the pull until you notice a fascial release.

Fascial Technique according to Finet and Williame

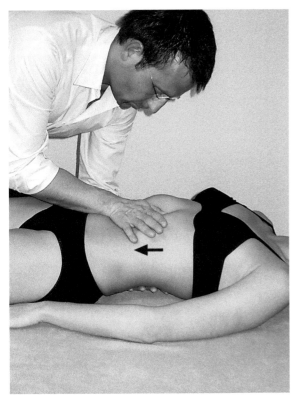

Fig. 10.4

Starting Position
The patient is in the supine position, legs stretched out. The practitioner stands on the patient's right side.

Procedure
Place your right hand on the projection of the pancreas with the heel of the hand on the head and the fingertips on the tail. Place your left hand on the posterior projection of the pancreas with the heel of the hand on the head and the fingertips on the tail.

Treatment
During inhalation, pull caudally with both hands at the same time; during exhalation hold the position reached. Repeat this procedure until you have reached the end of the fascial movement. In the next exhalation, release the pull.

Repeat the whole treatment four or five times.

Circulatory Techniques according to Kuchera

Arterial Stimulation

- stimulation of the celiac trunk and superior mesenteric artery by working on the spinal column
- diaphragm techniques

Venous Stimulation

- liver pump
- stretching the hepatoduodenal ligament
- diaphragm techniques

Lymphatic Stimulation

- lymph drainage on thorax and abdomen
- diaphragm techniques

Vegetative Harmonization

Sympathetic nervous system:
Stimulation of the sympathetic trunk T5–T9 by:
- rib raising
- inhibiting the paravertebral muscles
- vibrations
- manipulations
- Maitland technique
- stimulation of the celiac plexus
- diaphragm techniques

Parasympathetic nervous system:
Stimulation of the vagus nerve by:
- craniosacral therapy
- laryngeal techniques
- thoracic techniques (recoil)
- diaphragm techniques

Reflex Point Treatment according to Chapman

Location

Anterior. Intercostal space between ribs 7 and 8 on the right side, near the rib cartilage.

Posterior. Between the two transverse processes of T7 and T8, halfway between the spinous process and the tip of the transverse process; present only on the right side!

Treatment Principle

Make contact with the reflex point. For this purpose, very gently place a finger on the point and press only lightly. Reflex points are often very sensitive, and it is therefore important to proceed with caution.

The finger remains on the point and treatment is by gentle rotations.

The anterior points are treated first, then the posterior points. Continue with the treatment until you have normalized the sensitivity or consistency of the point.

To conclude, check the anterior points once more. If you fail to notice any change, it is possible that the organ pathology is too great to be influenced quickly via the reflex points, or other dysfunctions are present that must be treated first.

Recommendations for the Patient

Dietary advice for diabetes mellitus:

- Avoid obesity.
- Reduce consumption of refined sugar.
- Preferably choose complex carbohydrates.
- Take vitamin C, E, and chromium (brewer's yeast) supplements.

11 The Peritoneum

Anatomy

General Facts

Function

- mechanical protection by means of impact-buffering fat
- vascular function
- immune defense

Location

Parietal Peritoneum

- diaphragmatic part: underside of the diaphragm
- posterior part:
  - covers the transversal fascia and is separated from the abdominal wall by the retroperitoneal space
  - located in the retroperitoneal space are the aorta, inferior vena cava, kidney, ureter, and adrenal glands; the ureter is attached to the peritoneum by its cover of connective tissue

- anterior part: covers the anterolateral abdominal wall and forms:
  - supravesical fossa
  - medial inguinal fossa
  - lateral inguinal fossa (= weak spots in the abdominal wall—hernia gates)
- inferior part: lines the sidewalls of the pelvic cavity and lies along the median line of the subperitoneal connective tissue. In the female pelvis, the peritoneum forms two deep pouches:
  - vesicouterine pouch
  - rectouterine pouch (pouch of Douglas)

Visceral Peritoneum

The visceral peritoneum lies (firmly) against the inside of the parietal peritoneum and the surfaces of the abdominal organs.

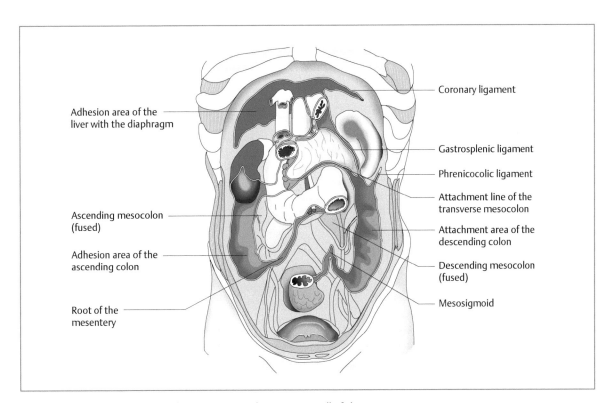

Fig. 11.1 Structures of the parietal peritoneum on the posterior wall of the torso.

Topographic Relationships

The peritoneum is topographically connected to all the intraperitoneal organs and to most of the retro- and extraperitoneal organs and structures.

Attachments/Suspensions

Mesenteries

The mesenteries attach the organs to the walls of the torso and supply them with vessels and nerves.

Mesentery of the Stomach

Gastropancreatic fold (with left gastric artery) with the duodenopancreatic ligament (with common hepatic artery)

Mesentery of the Small Intestine
- 12–15 cm long and 18 mm wide
- crosses L2–L5
- At the level L3–L4, the superior mesenteric vein enters the mesentery.
- Between L4 and L5, the mesentery crosses the right ureter.

The mesoappendix originates in the mesentery and continues into the appendico-ovarian ligament.

Transverse Mesocolon

The transverse mesocolon divides the peritoneal space into the upper and the lower abdomen.

Sigmoid Mesocolon
- One root runs vertically downward from the inferior mesenteric artery to S3.
- The second root of the sigmoid mesocolon runs diagonally from the inferior mesenteric artery to the inner edge of the left psoas.
- Additional connections exist to the left iliac artery, left fallopian tube, and mesentery.

The **ligament of Treitz** (suspensory muscle of the duodenum) runs from the crus of the diaphragm, the right edge of the esophagus, and the aortic hiatus to the duodenojejunal flexure.

The **Treitz fascia** constitutes the connection of the duodenum and the pancreas. In addition, it fixates the pancreas posteriorly onto the transversal fascia.

The **Toldt fascia** connects the ascending colon with the descending colon.

Both fasciae are the rudimentary embryonic mesenteries of these organs and point to their embryonic intraperitoneal location.

Ligaments

Ligaments connect two organs to each other or an organ to the wall of the abdomen, but do not contain important vessels. They include the:
- round ligament of the liver (ligamentum teres hepatis, obliterated umbilical vein)
- coronary ligament with left and right triangular ligaments
- gastrophrenic ligament (enveloping fold of the two leaves of the peritoneum that cover the stomach)—continues as the lesser omentum and gastrosplenic ligament
- broad ligament of the uterus (fixates the peritoneum firmly to the uterus and adnexas)
- phrenicocolic ligament (lateral continuation of the greater omentum)

Omenta

The omenta are infoldings of the peritoneum that sometimes contain vessels and run from one organ to another. They include the:
- lesser omentum
- greater omentum (a part of the greater omentum forms the gastrocolic ligament)
- gastrosplenic ligament (continuation of the gastrocolic ligament in a left-lateral direction)—continues on the inside of the spleen and as the anterior leaf of the pancreaticosplenic ligament
- pancreaticosplenic ligament (posterior short leaf continues as the posterior parietal peritoneum)

Omental Bursa

Borders
- at the back: posterior parietal peritoneum
- at the front: lesser omentum, stomach, transverse colon
- below: transverse mesocolon
- on the left: gastrosplenic and pancreaticosplenic ligaments

Circulation

The arterial, venous, and lymphatic circulations of the visceral peritoneum correspond to the supply lines of the organ. The parietal peritoneum is supplied segmentally.

Innervation

The peritoneum is supplied by sensory and vasomotor fibers from the phrenic nerve and the thoracic and lumbar segmental nerves.

Movement Physiology according to Barral

Motricity

As the parietal peritoneum is attached to the wall of the torso (see above), movements of the torso cause it to move as well, in the sense of stretching or approximating partial areas, e.g., if you lean the upper body backward, the anterior part of the peritoneum, which lies flat against the abdominal wall, is stretched. If postoperative adhesions are present, this can trigger pain.

A lateral flexion of the torso to the right approximates the right lateral part and stretches the left lateral part.

Mobility

The engine for this form of movement is the respiratory movement of the abdomen and diaphragm.

During inhalation, the respiratory movement in the diaphragm causes the entire peritoneal sac to shift caudally. In addition the subdiaphragmatic parts experience a shift medially in the lateral areas.

The abdominal wall is pushed anteriorly by the abdominal organs during inhalation; the peritoneum follows similarly. During exhalation, the opposite movement occurs.

Motility

If the peritoneum is not affected by dysfunctions, it carries out a rotation around a longitudinal axis. The right side rotates toward the right and the left side toward the left.

Physiology

Functions of the peritoneum and the greater omentum are:
- mechanical protection of the anterior abdominal wall
- immunological function by embedding numerous lymphatic cells and vessels, especially in the greater omentum
- Fat storage: the greater omentum can store considerable amounts of fat which could even cause a significant increase in abdominal pressure, with dysfunctions of the abdominal organs or diaphragm.

Pathologies

Symptoms that Require Medical Clarification

- Signs of peritonitis

Peritonitis

Definition. Acute or chronic inflammation of the peritoneum in local or diffuse/generalized form.

Causes
- infectious:
  - approximately 95 % of cases
  - perforation of a hollow organ
  - iatrogenic–postoperative
  - ascending from the fallopian tubes
- chemical–toxic:
  - bile
  - pancreatic secretion
  - urine
  - barium meal
  - foreign objects (suturing materials)
- induced by radiation

Clinical. Very strong persistent somatic pressure that develops progressively within seconds to hours spontaneously or from colic.
- rebound tenderness
- protective tension or rigidity
- first increased, later lacking intestinal sounds (paralytic icterus)
- abdominal distension
- dehydration
- shock

Osteopathic Practice

Cardinal Symptom

- Signs of peritonitis

Typical Dysfunctions

Adhesions/Fixations

- operations
- blunt trauma
- inflammation, e.g., appendicitis

Indications for Osteopathic Treatment

As the peritoneum lines the entire abdominal space and is connected topographically to all of the intraperitoneal and almost all of the retro- and extraperitoneal organs, the indications for treatment are extremely numerous.

Moreover, as it also belongs to the system of the "central tendon," fascial reactions in the peritoneum are also likely to be dysfunctions located further cranially or caudally.

A precise osteopathic analysis and thorough familiarity with the body's topography lead to the proper indication in each individual case.

Contraindications for Osteopathic Treatment

Acute Inflammation of the Peritoneum
This condition can arise locally as a concurrent reaction to an organ inflammation, e.g., appendicitis, or it can be generalized, e.g., in perforation of an appendix.

For symptoms of peritonitis, see page 105.

Notes for Clinical Application

As described in Chapter 17 (see page 187), the peritoneum is linked embryologically to the central tendon. In this function, it supports the body in constructing compensatory patterns to relieve stressed structures. For this task, the parietal peritoneum is of particular importance. Similar to a fully inflated air balloon, it lines the abdominal walls on all sides. It is able to transmit fascial tensions through all sides: in some cases, the body utilizes primarily the anterior parietal peritoneum, e.g., when a cesarean section scar must be protected; in other cases fascial tensions that originate in the diaphragm are conducted through the posterior peritoneum caudally. In this context, two features are noteworthy:
1. The posterior parietal peritoneum extends deeply into the lesser pelvis and, via the rectum and uterus, creates contact with the most caudal section of the central tendon, the lamina of Delbet (see page 156).
2. Anteriorly, there are bulges in the peritoneum that can be explained by embryology and degenerate after birth into ligaments. Here, we are referring to the medial and lateral umbilical ligaments, which are leftovers of the umbilical artery, and the median umbilical ligament, which runs from the tip of the bladder to the navel. The other two ligaments come out of the depths of the lesser pelvis, pass to the right and left of the bladder, and end at the navel as well. From there, the round ligament of the liver runs cranially. It constitutes the obliterated remainder of the umbilical vein and forms the caudal edge of the falciform ligament, which turns into the coronary ligament of the liver and ends at the diaphragm. In this way, continuity

from the diaphragm to the lesser pelvis is ensured by anterior structures as well.

It should be mentioned that the peritoneum is connected to all intra-, retro-, and extraperitoneal organs either directly or via other fasciae. It can respond to dysfunctions in the organs by fascially contracting as part of the central tendon in such a way that the organ is protected (see page 7). As a result of its connection to all the abdominal organs, it is very common to detect abnormal tensions in the peritoneum.

On the other hand, it is also possible for peritoneal tensions that originated in the peritoneum, as part of the mechanism of the central tendon, to be conveyed to other organs, thereby causing an osteopathic dysfunction in these organs.

Detailed examination of the organs and peritoneal tension is therefore indispensable for deciding whether we should treat the organ or the central tendon.

Osteopathic Tests and Treatment

Test and Treatment of Mobility according to Barral

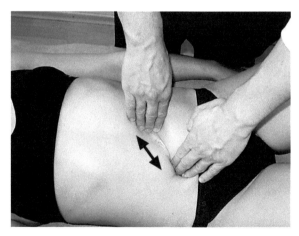

Fig. 11.2

Starting Position
The patient is in the supine position, legs stretched out. The practitioner stands next to the patient.

Procedure
Place both hands on the abdomen and push posteriorly until you have reached the correct palpatory plane for the peritoneum. (The correct plane: if you feel the organs, you have gone too deep. Withdraw out of the abdomen a little just to the point where you no longer feel, for example, the intestinal loops.)

Testing Sequence

One hand now becomes the punctum fixum, the other the punctum mobile. With the mobile hand, stretch the peritoneum around the fixed hand. In side-by-side comparison, evaluate local differences in tension and sensitivities to pulling. Proceed across the entire abdomen in this way and examine the entire anterior peritoneum. You can then switch the fixed and mobile hands.

Treatment

Locations with increased tension or sensitive areas are treated directly (by stretching the tissue) or indirectly (by converging the tissue). You can switch the fixed hand, or you can use both hands as mobile hands.

Variation

You can also select a seated position as your starting position.

Test and Treatment of Motility according to Barral

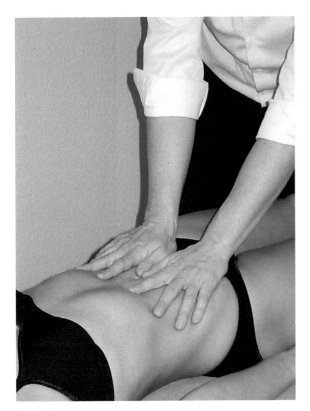

Fig. 11.3

Starting Position

The patient is in the supine position, legs stretched out. The practitioner stands next to the patient.

Procedure

Place both hands with fingers spread apart without pressure on the abdomen, to the right and left of the median line. If no disturbances are present, you can detect supination movement in the hands.

Testing Sequence

Find the motility motion and evaluate the amplitude and direction of the inspiratory and expiratory movements, as well as the rhythm of the movement as a whole. If a disturbance is present in one or both aspects of the motility movement, treat the patient.

Treatment

Motility is treated indirectly by following the unimpaired movement, remaining at the end-point of this movement for several cycles, and then following the impaired movement to the new end-point.

You can also try to increase the range of the free movement (induction), afterward checking whether the limited movement direction has improved.

Repeat this movement again and again until the motility has returned to normal in terms of rhythm, direction, and amplitude.

Local Listening Test

Starting Position

The patient is in the supine position, legs stretched out. The practitioner stands next to the patient.

Procedure

Place one hand on the abdomen on top of the navel. Apply just enough pressure posteriorly to reach the correct palpatory plane (see above). Now find the fascial movement and follow it. The area to which the hand is drawn is the location of increased tension (diagnostic zone). Then you can again place the hand in this area to further differentiate the exact location: when you have arrived at the place of greatest tension, you will no longer detect any fascial movement—this is where you need to treat.

Indirect Mobilization of the Peritoneum
with Long Arm Lever according to Barral

General Relief Technique according to Barral

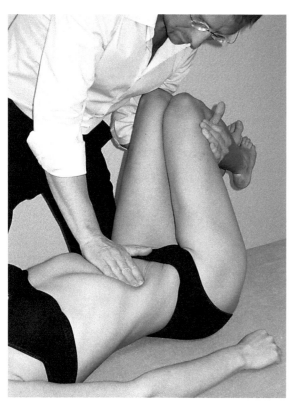

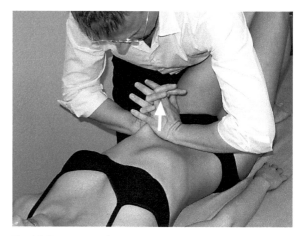

Fig. 11.5

Starting Position
The patient is in the supine position, legs bent. The practitioner stands next to the patient.

Procedure
With a pinch grip, grasp the entire abdominal wall including the peritoneum and carefully stretch all structures anteriorly. In this way, a pulling sensation may arise all the way to the spinal column. Hold this pull for up to 1 min. You can also apply this grip to individual areas of the peritoneum.

This technique is very effective but must be applied with caution because it can be very painful.

Variation
You can choose the "knee–elbow stand" as an alternative starting position. The advantage here is the good relaxation of the abdominal wall. The pinch grip is applied and executed in the same way.

Fig. 11.4

Starting Position
The patient is in the supine position, legs stretched out. The practitioner stands next to the patient.

Procedure
With the cranial hand, fixate the peritoneum. The caudal hand holds the legs in the knee bend and guides them in such a way that the fixed peritoneal area is stretched.

The stretch can be performed as a continuous pull or dynamically.

Variation
In a seated starting position, fixate an area of the peritoneum with the caudal hand. The patient interlocks the hands behind the neck. Now take hold of the patient's elbow with your cranial hand and guide it into an extension and rotation until the fixated peritoneal area is stretched.

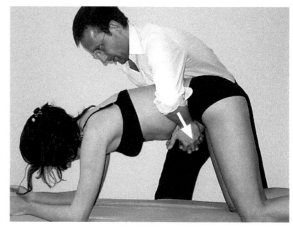

Fig. 11.6

Mobilization of the Posterior Peritoneum according to Roussé

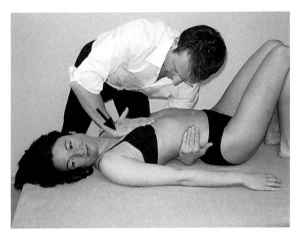

Fig. 11.7

Mobilization of the Caudal Peritoneum according to Roussé

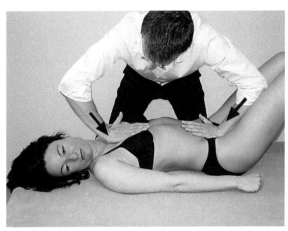

Fig. 11.8

Starting Position
The patient is in the supine position, legs stretched out. The practitioner stands next to the patient.

Procedure
Place your cranial hand onto the lower third of the sternum, with the forearm resting on the sternum. With the caudal hand, embrace the abdomen from posterior at the height of the lumbar spinal column so that your hand lies on the patient's contralateral flank and the upper arm on the equilateral flank.

With the cranial arm, apply pressure in a caudal–posterior direction while at the same time pressing the hand and upper arm of the caudal arm toward each other. These movements are combined with respiration: during exhalation, increase the pressure; during inhalation, hold the reached pressure. Repeat this procedure three or four times until you suddenly release the pressure at the start of an inhalation.

Starting Position
The patient is in the supine position, legs bent. The practitioner stands next to the patient.

Procedure
Position the cranial hand as shown in **Fig. 11.7**. Place the caudal hand on top of the pubis.

During exhalation, apply pressure with the cranial arm in a caudal–posterior direction. With the caudal hand, give a push cranially. Hold the position reached during inhalation and then increase the pressure again with the next exhalation. Repeat this procedure three or four times until you suddenly release the pressure at the start of an inhalation.

You can also place the caudal hand at the inner edge of the iliac wing. The mobilizing push is now applied in a cranial–medial direction.

12 The Jejunum and Ileum

Anatomy

General Facts

The total length of the jejunum/ileum is 5–6 m, of which two-fifths is the jejunum and three-fifths the ileum. This section of the small intestine starts at the duodenojejunal flexure and ends at the ileocecal valve, where it runs into the cecum.

Location

Arrangement of the small intestine is into 15–16 loops, the jejunum more horizontal and the ileum more vertical. Furthermore, the jejunum is located more around the navel, while the ileum is found in the right lower abdomen. As a whole, the jejunum and ileum lie more on the left side: the loops cover the descending colon while the ascending colon remains exposed.

Root of the Mesentery

The root of the mesentery is approximately 12–15 cm long and 18 mm wide. It extends from the duodenojejunal flexure to the ileocecal valve and so crosses L2–L5 in a diagonal course.

At the level of L3–L4, the superior mesenteric vein enters the mesentery. Between L4 and L5, the root crosses the ureter on the right side. The mesoappendix originates in the mesentery and continues into the appendico-ovarian ligament. At its distal end, the root crosses the testicular/ovarian vein.

Topographic Relationships

Anterior and Cranial

- transverse colon
- transverse mesocolon
- greater omentum
- anterior abdominal wall

Posterior

- posterior parietal peritoneum
- kidneys
- ureter
- aorta
- inferior vena cava
- common iliac vein
- duodenum
- descending and ascending colon

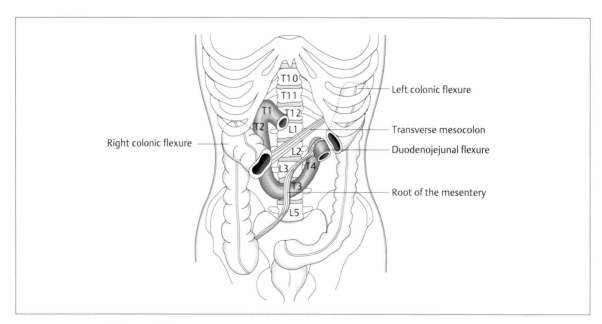

Fig. 12.1 Location of the root of the mesentery.

Caudal

- bladder
- uterus
- rectum

Lateral

- ascending colon
- abdominal wall
- cecum
- sigmoid colon

Attachments/Suspensions

- organ pressure
- turgor
- root of the mesentery

Circulation

Arterial

Superior mesenteric artery.

Venous

Portal vein.

Lymph Drainage

Along the vessels to the superior mesenteric lymph nodes —celiac and lumbar lymph nodes.

Innervation

- sympathetic nervous system from T10 to T12 via the minor splanchnic nerve to the superior mesenteric ganglion
- vagus nerve

Organ Clock

Maximal time: 1–3 p. m.
Minimal time: 1–3 a.m.

Organ–Tooth Interrelationship

For basic information, see page 34.

- Wisdom tooth in the lower jaw on both sides

Movement Physiology according to Barral

Mobility

The diaphragm has only a minor effect on this area of the small intestine. Nevertheless, we can deduce from the type of suspension that large movements must be taking place in the jejunum and ileum. These are the intrinsic movements necessary for mixing the food mash and propelling the chyme (peristalsis).

Motility

In the expiratory phase, the entire bundle of the small intestine performs a clockwise rotation; during the inspiratory phase, it goes back in the opposite direction.

Physiology

Microscopic Wall Structure

In these sections of the intestine, we find the typical wall structure of the entire digestive tract (esophagus to rectum).
  The layers are:
- mucous membrane
- tela submucosa
- muscular layer
- adventitia
- serosa

Mucous Membrane (Mucosa)

- epithelium
- lamina propria mucosae (reticular connective tissue)
- lamina muscularis mucosae (smooth muscle)

The inner surface of the intestine feels smooth like velvet. This is the result of the 0.5–1-mm high fingerlike projections into the mucosa (villi), which are arranged close to each other in evenly spaced intervals. At the base of these villi, we find the tubular phlegm-producing glands of the intestines (crypts) which sink deeply from this base into the depth.
  The epithelial cells of the villi are furthermore marked by evaginations in the membrane (ciliated border, microvilli), which increase the surface of the intestine, as well as the villi and crypts, by many times: the inner surface of the intestine thereby reaches almost twice the size of the surface of the skin ($4 m^2$).
  The villi are the site of absorption, and the crypts the site of regeneration and secretion. Diverse food particles are absorbed by the greatly enlarged surface of the villi, whereas the crypt cells provide for the renewal of dead epithelial cells and of the mucus that covers the inner surface of the intestine.

Tela Submucosa

The tela submucosa consists of connective tissue. It includes:
- the Meissner plexus (submucous plexus), which supplies the smooth muscle and the glands
- circulation for the mucosa
- the Peyer patches (lymph follicles that increase in number distally)

Mucosa and submucosa form the circular crossfolds of the intestine (valves of Kerckring = plicae circulares), which are visible with the naked eye. They serve to enlarge the surface area and decrease in number distally.

Muscular Layer

The muscular layer consists of smooth muscle cells that are arranged in an inner ring-shaped and an outer longitudinal muscle layer. The peristaltic and chyme-mixing movements originate in these muscles.

In a layer of connective tissue between these two layers, we find the Auerbach plexus (myenteric plexus), which supplies the two muscular layers vegetatively.

Adventitia

The adventitia is a layer of connective tissue that is very pronounced in those areas of the intestine that are not covered by peritoneum. In the area of the jejunum and ileum, this layer is therefore only very thin and called subserosa.

Serosa

This is the visceral peritoneum.

Regional Differences in Wall Structure between the Jejunum and Ileum

Jejunum. In the proximal parts of the jejunum, the valves of Kerckring and villi are very dense, and the ciliated border contains a particularly large quantity of enzymes: most of the absorptive processes for carbohydrates, fats, and proteins occur in the first 100 cm of the jejunum. Distally, the valves of Kerckring decrease in number and height, but we find more lymphatic follicles.

Ileum. Distally, the valves of Kerckring disappear completely; instead, we find a large number of Peyer patches, which are involved in immune defense.

Processes of Absorption in the Jejunum and Ileum

These two sections of the intestine are the main location for the digestion and absorption of fats, carbohydrates, proteins, vitamins, inorganic salts, and water. The digestive enzymes produced by the small intestine are located partly in the ciliated border on the lumen side; others are spread diffusely in the cytoplasm of the epithelial cells and released only after the cells die off. The short lifespan of the cells in the intestinal mucosa, i.e., 2–3 days, accommodates this physiology.

Each day, the body absorbs 8–9 L of water with 50–100 g electrolytes in the small intestine, but of these only 1.5 L comes from food; the rest is discharged as digestive secretions from the intestine.

Digestion of Carbohydrates

The α-amylase in the saliva and pancreas breaks starch down into oligosaccharides. Together with disaccharides from food, these are further broken down by enzymes in the ciliated border into monosaccharides and in this form absorbed by the membrane.

Digestion of Fats

With the assistance of bile salts, lipases in the saliva and pancreas split triglycerides in the food into monoglycerides and free fatty acids. In combination with the products of fat digestion and fat-soluble vitamins, the bile salts form micelles. Micelles attach themselves to the epithelium of the small intestine and mediate the absorption of the products of fat digestion into the mucous membrane. The bile salts themselves are entered into an enterohepatic cycle in the terminal ileum.

Digestion of Proteins

The acid gastric juice denatures the proteins in the food—it dismantles the three-dimensional structure of proteins. Pepsins in the gastric juice then split the proteins into medium–long and short peptides. The pancreatic enzymes (trypsin and chymotrypsin) further cleave the proteins into oligopeptides, which are then broken down by enzymes in the ciliated border into amino acids, or di- or tripeptides, and absorbed by the mucosa in the small intestine.

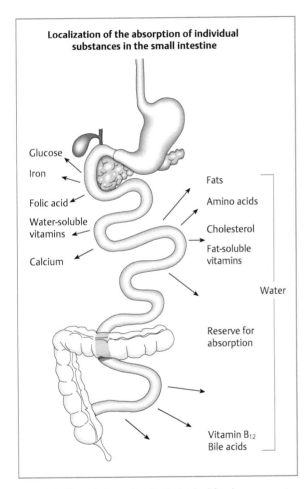

Fig. 12.2 Sites of absorption for individual food components.

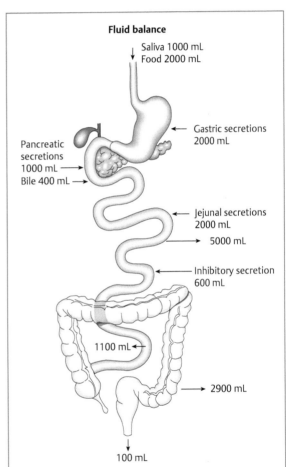

Fig. 12.3 Fluid balance.

Pathologies

Symptoms that Require Medical Clarification

> • Bloody stools
> • Diarrhea that persists for more than 5 days
> • Signs of peritonitis

Crohn Disease

Definition. Chronic inflammation of the intestinal walls. The inflammation can affect all wall layers. The terminal ileum and colon are affected most frequently, but it is also possible that the entire gastrointestinal tract is infected.

Causes. The cause is unknown; familial aggregation has been observed.

Clinical. The symptoms arise periodically and in connection with the activity of the inflammatory process.
• abnormal abdominal pain
• three to six bowel movements with soft stools per day, also at night
• weight loss
• fever
• elevated erythrocyte sedimentation rate
• perianal fistulae as a precursor of Crohn disease
• most common complications:
  – fistulae
  – abscesses
  – stenoses

Crohn disease can simulate the symptoms of acute appendicitis.

Celiac Disease/Sprue

Definition. Allergy to gluten in European types of grain, which leads to villous atrophy and malabsorption.

Causes. Gluten intolerance.

Clinical
• increased stool weight, one to four bowel movements per day, steatorrhea
• lactose intolerance
• malabsorption with deficiency of trace elements and vitamins, as well as impaired growth and failure to thrive, e.g.:
  – osteomalacia
  – tetany
  – bleeding tendency
  – dystrophy of the hair and skin

– protein deficiency edema
– being underweight

Osteopathic Practice

Cardinal Symptoms

> • Periumbilical pain and cramping
> • Bloody stools

Typical Dysfunctions

• adhesions/fixations
• ptosis
• spasms

Associated Structural Dysfunctions

T10–L2.

Atypical Symptoms

A list of symptoms follows that can be explained by means of osteopathic chains or result from the patient's history (for an explanation of osteopathic chains, see "Atypical Symptoms" in Chapter 5, page 39):
• disturbing pulling sensation below the navel approximately 3–4 hours after meals
• discomfort when wearing tight pants or belts
• lumbago after standing for longer periods of time
• difficulty breathing, especially during exhalation, after standing for longer periods of time
• visible ptosis, often in combination with a hypomobile cervicothoracic junction ("widow's hump")
• asthenic patients have a greater tendency to problems in the small intestines (ptosis)

Indications for Osteopathic Treatment

Adhesions/Fixations

These can arise after any surgical intervention in the abdominal area. The loops of the small intestine can adhere to each other or to other organs, or individual loops can grow together with the anterior abdominal wall.

Another cause can be inflammatory diseases: Crohn disease, acute gastroenteritis, and appendicitis are some of the possible pathologies for which healing processes must be completed before we can apply treatment.

Ptosis of the entire bundle of the small intestine as the result of gravity can be observed along the root of the mesentery in the left lower abdomen. Similarly, small intestinal loops can migrate into the lesser pelvis if they find enough space there, e.g., after removal of the uterus.

Occlusions can be the cause of ptosis in the small intestine. In recurrent diverticulitis, for example, adhesions/fixations can form in the left lower abdomen which lead to connective tissue pulling on the intestinal loops in a left–downward direction.

Other reasons for a ptosis of the jejunum and ileum include:
- scars from surgery
- retroversion of the uterus
- lower abdominal surgery with organ removal
- childbirth
- hormonal relaxation of the connective tissue after pregnancy
- age-related loss of tonicity in the tissue
- asthenic body

Contraindications for Osteopathic Treatment

- acute inflammations
- fever
- new scars
- bloody stools
- signs of peritonitis

Notes for Clinical Application

In the entire gastrointestinal tract there are more nerve cells than in the spinal cord. For the most part, the autonomy of this nervous system takes place with no conscious perception: normally, we do not feel any of the peristalsis in the stomach or intestines, even though there is continuous movement in our abdomen—an automatic action that works for us without ever being noticed by us.

In spite of the fact that the intestines thus work imperceptibly, we nevertheless have a special relationship to our "abdominal brain." Numerous colloquial expressions provide evidence for this fact, e.g.:
- "He can stomach anything."
- "It makes my stomach turn."
- "I had butterflies in my stomach."
- "I trust my gut feeling."
- "This made me sick to my stomach!"

These emotional expressions related to the gastrointestinal tract account for the fact that a disorder of the intestines or stomach is experienced as very distressing and stifling. Often, we feel even more sick than in a truly life-threatening condition such as a heart attack, in which we can feel almost completely recovered after a few days of convalescence, even though we are still acutely at risk of death.

We thus have a special relationship to our belly and its innards. That this connection can also be used by our body to shift psychological stress situations into the physical arena can be seen in the fact that the intestines or stomach often run wild before examinations; irritable colon and irritable bowel are technical expressions for such conditions.

Nevertheless, the intestine is a defense organ. In the ileum, we find a profusion of lymphatic cells that aggregate in the appendix to form thick lymph follicles, as a result of which it is also called the "intestinal tonsil." These Peyer patches have an important immunological function to fulfill, because our food includes a large number of protein molecules that can also act as antigens. In addition, we naturally ingest a multitude of virulent organisms in our food, which can be intercepted here.

Thus, on the one hand, the intestine is a defense organ and, on the other, we have a special psychological relationship to our belly. Both aspects can coincide, with unfortunate results: there are many patients with a disturbed immune defense in the intestines, resulting in numerous food allergies. These hyperallergenic periods are not permanent, but linked to stressful phases of life. Afterwards, they disappear again.

Osteopathic Tests and Treatment

Test and Treatment of the Intestinal Loops in the Supine Position according to Barral

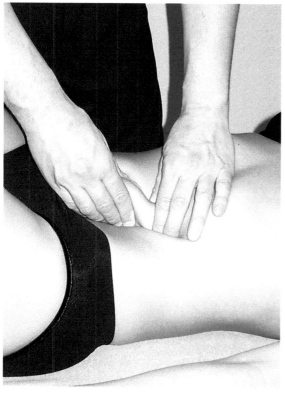

Fig. 12.4

Test for Ptosis of the Small Intestine in the Seated or Standing Position according to Barral

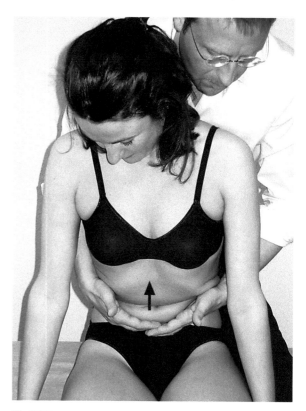

Fig. 12.5

Starting Position

The patient is in the supine position, legs bent. The practitioner stands next to the patient.

Procedure

Sink both hands into the abdomen at the level of the navel and palpate the small intestinal loops for differences in tonus (spasms) and sensitivities. In this way, cover the entire area where the loops are located: around the navel, laterally (especially to the left), and in the entire lower abdominal region.

Treatment

The loops that are sensitive or marked by elevated tonicity are stretched, inhibited, or gently wrung against each other until you have normalized the tonus or reduced the pain.

Starting Position

The patient sits or stands. The practitioner stands in front of or behind the patient.

Procedure

Lift the entire bundle of the small intestine with both hands as far as it will go and then abruptly let it fall back down.

Evaluation

If the action of letting it fall is painful or triggers the typical pain in the patient, this is an indication that the jejunum/ileum is involved.

Test and Treatment of the Mesenteric Root in the Side Position according to Barral

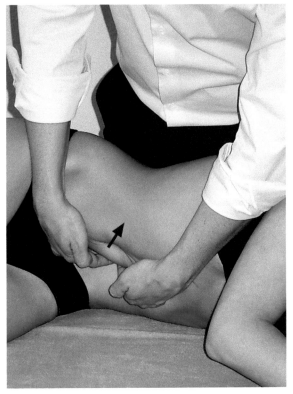

Fig. 12.6

Starting Position
The patient is in the lateral position facing left, legs bent. The practitioner stands behind the patient.

Procedure
With both hands next to each other, reach into the abdomen lateral to the small intestinal loops and medial to the descending colon. The loops now lie in your palms, the direction of palpation being in a posteromedial direction. In this way, reach the root of the mesentery deep down, in its slanted course from left top to right bottom. Now palpate its entire length for differences in tonicity and sensitivities, thereby stretching it in the direction of the patient's right shoulder.

Treatment
If differences in tonicity or sensitivities are found, stretch the root in the direction of the patient's right shoulder with a constant pull until the symptoms are clearly reduced or disappear completely. You can apply this treatment over the entire length of the root or at isolated spots.

Variation
The area around the ileocecal valve can also be treated as follows. Visualize the course of the root and, from the same starting position, reach into the abdomen from medial to the cecum. Both hands lie next to each other, with the intestinal loops on the backs of the fingers. Once you reach the root from the right, mobilize it in the direction of the left iliac wing.

The area around the ileocecal valve tends to be very sensitive; we must therefore use extra caution.

General Relief Technique of the Peritoneum and Intestinal Loops in the Supine Position according to Barral

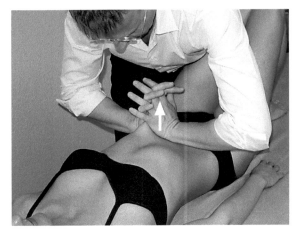

Fig. 12.7

Starting Position
The patient is in the supine position, legs bent. The practitioner stands next to the patient.

Procedure
With a pinch grip, grasp the entire abdominal wall, including the peritoneum, and carefully stretch all structures anteriorly. In this way, a pulling sensation may arise all the way to the spinal column. Hold this pull for up to 1 min. You can also apply this grip to individual areas of the peritoneum.

This technique is very effective for adhesions/fixations but must be applied with caution because it can be very painful.

If you apply the grip slightly further posteriorly into the abdomen, you capture part of the small intestinal loops as well.

The anterior pull can thus also include the root of the mesentery.

Variation

You can choose the "knee–elbow stand" as an alternative starting position. The advantage here is the good relaxation of the abdominal wall. The pinch grip is applied and executed in the same way.

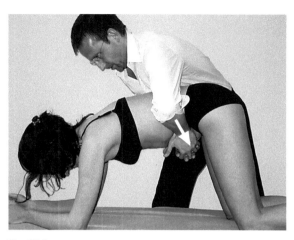

Fig. 12.8

Treatment of Intestinal Ptosis

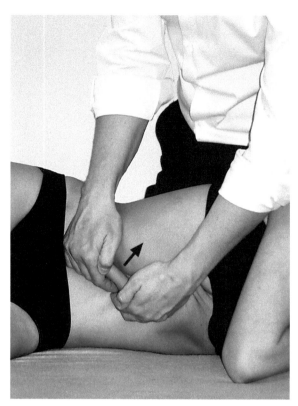

Fig. 12.9

Starting Position

The patient is in the lateral position facing left, legs bent. The practitioner stands behind the patient.

Procedure

With both hands, grasp the entire bundle of the intestines and mobilize in the direction of the patient's right shoulder, with a continuous pull or intermittently.

The aim of this technique is not to return the ptotic intestine to its old location but to provide it with the greatest possible freedom to move on its new gliding surface.

Variation

Other starting positions are possible. For self-mobilization, the supine position with elevated pelvis is especially suitable.

Treatment of the Ileocecal Valve according to Barral

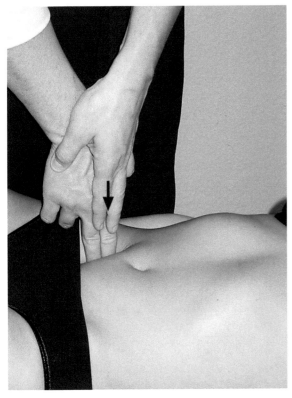

Fig. 12.10

Starting Position
The patient is in the supine position, legs stretched out. The practitioner stands on the patient's right side.

Procedure
To find the ileocecal valve, you have to look for its approximate projection onto the abdominal wall. For this purpose, draw a line from the right anterosuperior iliac spine (ASIS) to the navel and divide it into thirds. At the transition from the lateral to the middle third, place your fingers on the abdominal wall. Now slide slowly posteriorly into the abdomen. You should proceed slowly in order to give the superficially located structures time to move out of the way and allow for fascial relaxation.

Once you have advanced deeply enough in this palpation, you will find a supple, roughly hazelnut-sized solidification within 0.5–1 cm of this palpation point. In most cases, the ileocecal valve is sensitive to palpation.

You can now apply small circulations, vibrations, or inhibitions, until the tonicity or sensitivity is clearly reduced.

Test and Treatment of Motility according to Barral

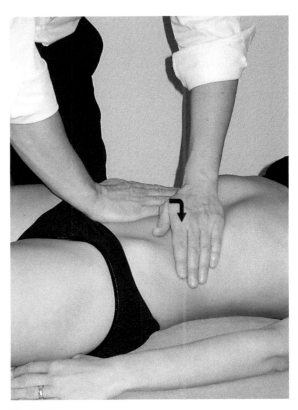

Fig. 12.11

Starting Position
The patient is in the supine position, legs stretched out. The practitioner stands on the patient's right side.

Procedure
Place the cranial hand without pressure to the left of the median line on the area of the horizontal small intestinal loops, with the fingertips pointing in a left-lateral direction. Place the caudal hand, also without pressure, to the right of the median line on the area of the vertical loops, with the fingertips pointing caudally.

Testing Sequence
Detect the motility movement: in the expiratory phase, the entire bundle of the small intestine performs a clockwise rotation; during the inspiratory phase, it moves back in the opposite direction. Evaluate the amplitude and direction of the inspiratory and expiratory movements as well as the rhythm of the movement as a whole. If a disturbance is present in one or both aspects of the motility movement, treat the patient.

Treatment

Motility is treated indirectly by following the unimpaired movement, remaining at the end-point of this movement for several cycles, and then following the impaired movement to the new end-point.

You can also try to increase the range of the free movement (induction), afterward checking whether the limited movement direction has improved.

Repeat this movement again and again until the motility has returned to normal in terms of rhythm, direction, and amplitude.

Fascial Treatment according to Finet and Williame

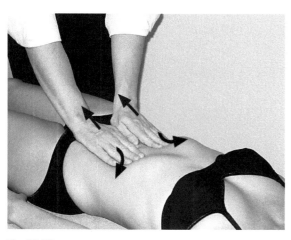

Fig. 12.12

Starting Position

The patient is in the supine position, legs stretched out. The practitioner stands by the patient's right side.

Procedure

Place both hands on the abdomen, one hand to the right and the other to the left of the median line. The fingertips point cranially. With both hands, apply just enough pressure posteriorly to reach the fascial plane.

Treatment

During inhalation, pull with both hands simultaneously caudally and rotate with the fingertips away from each other (the right hand clockwise, the left hand counterclockwise). During exhalation, maintain the position reached. Repeat this procedure until you have reached the end of the fascial movement. In the next exhalation, release the pull.

Repeat the whole treatment four or five times.

Circulatory Techniques according to Kuchera

Arterial Stimulation

- stimulation of the superior mesenteric artery by working on the spinal column
- diaphragm techniques

Venous Stimulation

- liver pump
- stretching the hepatoduodenal ligament
- diaphragm techniques

Lymphatic Stimulation

- lymph drainage on thorax and abdomen
- diaphragm techniques

Vegetative Harmonization

Sympathetic nervous system:
Stimulation of the sympathetic trunk T10–T12 by:
- rib raising
- inhibiting the paravertebral muscles
- vibrations
- manipulations
- Maitland technique
- stimulating the superior mesenteric ganglion
- diaphragm techniques

Parasympathetic nervous system:
Stimulation of the vagus nerve by:
- craniosacral therapy
- laryngeal techniques
- thoracic techniques (recoil)
- diaphragm techniques

Reflex Point Treatment according to Chapman

Location

Anterior. Intercostal spaces between ribs 8 and 9, 9 and 10, and 10 and 11 near the rib cartilage (on both sides).

Posterior. Between the two transverse processes of T8–T9, T9–T10, and T10–T11, halfway between the spinous process and the tip of the transverse process (on both sides).

Principle

Make contact with the reflex point. For this purpose, very gently place a finger on the point and press only lightly. Reflex points are often very sensitive, so it is important to proceed with caution.

The finger remains on the point and treatment is by gentle rotations.

The anterior points are treated first, then the posterior points. Continue with the treatment until you have normalized the sensitivity or consistency of the point.

To conclude, check the anterior points once more. If you fail to notice any change, it is possible that the organ pathology is too great to be influenced quickly via the reflex points, or other dysfunctions are present that must be treated first.

Recommendations for the Patient

- Consume only small amounts of industrially processed carbohydrates.
- Preferably select foods rich in fiber.
- Protein-rich foods (meat, cheese) should be avoided as much as possible in the evening.

Self-Treatment of a Ptosis

Supine position with head down and self-mobilization of the intestinal bundle cranially.

13 The Colon

Anatomy

General Facts

Length: approximately 1.5 m
  Diameter:
- ascending colon 7–8 cm
- transverse colon 5 cm
- descending colon 3–5 cm
- sigmoid colon 3–5 cm

Significant angles:
- hepatic flexure (right colic flexure)
- splenic flexure (left colic flexure)
- ileocecal valve
- sigmoid angle

Special characteristics:
- no villi and mucous membrane folds, only crypts
- semilunar folds (contracted ring muscles, not constant)
- haustra (noncontracted sections of the intestine)
- taeniae coli (strong bands of longitudinal muscle, run together into a continuous muscle layer at the appendix and sigmoid)

- epiploic appendices (small pouches of serosa filled with fat)

Location

Cecum

- intraperitoneal
- Runs diagonally in a caudal–medial–anterior direction and ends at the right iliac fossa.
- approximately 7 cm long
- The ileocecal valve is found on the left side (superior and slightly posterior).

Vermiform Appendix

- 5–10 cm long
- variability in diverse locations
- projection onto the wall of the torso: approximately 2 cm superior to McBurney point

Ascending Colon

- retroperitoneal
- pathway: on the right side in the lateral region superiorly and slightly posteriorly

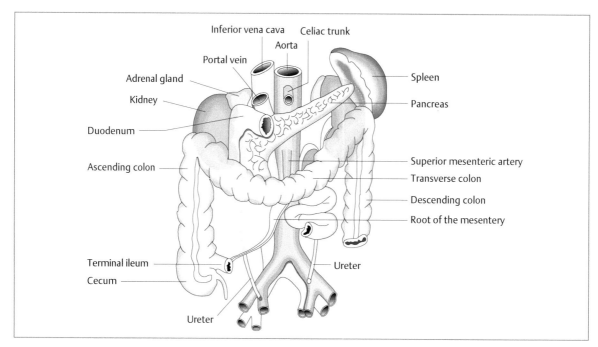

Fig. 13.1 Location of the colon.

Right Colic Flexure

- angle of 70–80°
- oriented sagittally with the opening in an anterior–caudal–medial direction
- projection onto the wall of the torso: rib 10 anterior to the right

Transverse Colon

- intraperitoneal
- The left end lies higher than the right end.
- Has a concave shape posteriorly.
- Location is variable. We usually find it between two horizontal lines—one going through the ninth costal cartilage and the other through the navel—but it also extends to the lesser pelvis.

Left Colic Flexure

- greater mobility than the right flexure
- angle of 50°
- frontosagittal orientation with the opening in an anteromedial direction
- projection: eighth rib anterior to the left

Descending Colon

- retroperitoneal
- lies further posteriorly than the ascending colon in the lateral area on the left

Sigmoid Colon

- intraperitoneal
- Runs from the posterosuperior part of the iliac fossa along the outer edge of the left psoas, crosses it 3–4 cm in front of the inguinal ligament, enters the lesser pelvis, and ends at the height of S3 in the rectum.
- Middle section can have a diameter of 15 cm.
- Pelvic section of the sigmoid can be displaced upward by a full bladder, the rectum, its own state of fullness, or the uterus.

Proximal Rectum

Retroperitoneal.

Distal Rectum

Extraperitoneal.

Topographic Relationships

Cecum

- abdominal wall
- posterior peritoneum
- iliac fascia
- iliacus
- envelope of the external iliac artery and vein
- inguinal ligament
- psoas major
- lateral cutaneous nerve of the thigh
- femoral nerve
- genitofemoral nerve
- small intestinal loops

Vermiform Appendix

- right ovary
- possible contact with the bladder, rectum, and uterus

Ascending Colon

- iliac fossa
- covered by peritoneum
- right kidney
- Toldt fascia
- subcostal nerve
- iliohypogastric nerve
- ilioinguinal nerve
- aponeurosis of quadratus lumborum, kidney fascia, iliac fascia
- lateral and anterior abdominal wall
- diaphragm
- small intestinal loops
- duodenum (descending part)
- liver
- rib 11

Right Colic Flexure

- liver
- duodenum (descending part)
- diaphragm
- right kidney
- phrenicocolic ligament on the right

Transverse Colon

- liver
- gallbladder
- abdominal wall indirectly via the greater omentum
- greater curvature of the stomach

Transverse Mesocolon

- pancreas
- duodenum
- jejunum
- left kidney
- spleen

Left Colic Flexure

- greater curvature of the stomach
- spleen
- phrenicocolic ligament on the left
- diaphragm
- lateral abdominal wall
- rib 8/9

Descending Colon

- covered by peritoneum
- left kidney
- small intestinal loops
- Toldt fascia
- posterior abdominal wall
- subcostal nerve
- iliohypogastric nerve
- ilioinguinal nerve
- rib 10/11

Sigmoid Colon

- iliac fascia
- Toldt fascia
- iliacus
- small intestinal loops
- lateral cutaneous nerve of the thigh
- rectum
- uterus
- left ovary and fallopian tube

Sigmoid Mesocolon

- left ureter
- testicular/ovarian vessels on the left
- external iliac vein

Attachments/Suspensions

- turgor
- organ pressure

Cecum

- posterior peritoneum (superior part)
- mesentery (inferior part)

Ascending Colon

- peritoneum
- Toldt fascia

Right Colic Flexure

- peritoneum
- phrenicocolic ligament
- hepatocolic ligament (from the liver via the flexure to the right kidney)
- cystoduodenal ligament (extension of the hepatoduodenal ligament)

Transverse Colon

- transverse mesocolon
- greater omentum (ends at the phrenicocolic ligaments)
- gastrocolic ligament (part of the greater omentum): as a result of this ligament, the right part of the transverse colon has greater mobility

Left Colic Flexure

Phrenicocolic ligament.

Descending Colon

Toldt fascia.

Sigmoid Colon

Sigmoid mesocolon.

Circulation

Arterial

- superior mesenteric artery
- inferior mesenteric artery

Venous

Portal vein.

Lymph Drainage

- superior mesenteric lymph nodes
- celiac lymph nodes
- lumbar lymph nodes
- inferior mesenteric lymph nodes
- left lumbar lymphatic trunk

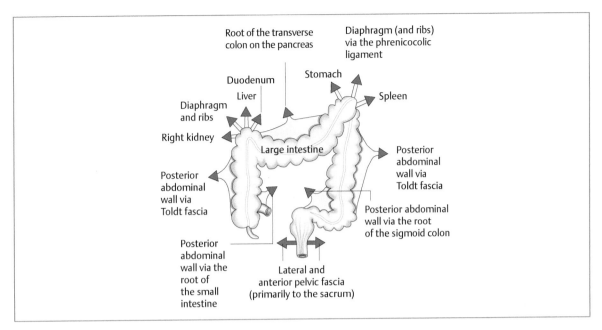

Fig. 13.2 Attachments of the colon, schematic.

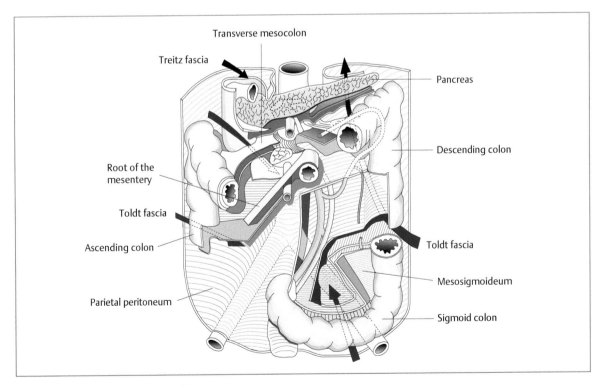

Fig. 13.3 Mesenteric attachments of the colon.

Innervation

- sympathetic nervous system from T10 to L2 via the greater and lesser splanchnic nerves
- T10–T11 via the superior mesenteric ganglion
- T12–L2 via the inferior mesenteric ganglion
- parasympathetic nervous system
- vagus nerve (ends at the superior mesenteric ganglion)

Sacral parasympathetic innervation from S2 to S4 via:
- pelvic splanchnic nerves–inferior hypogastric plexus–hypogastric nerves
- superior hypogastric plexus–inferior mesenteric plexus

Organ Clock

Maximal time: 5–7 a.m.
Minimal time: 5–7 p.m.

Organ–Tooth Interrelationship

For basic information, see page 34.

- First molar in the lower jaw on the right for the right colon
- First molar in the lower jaw on the left for the left colon
- First back tooth in the upper jaw on the left for the left colon
- First back tooth in the upper jaw on the right for the right colon

Movement Physiology according to Barral

Mobility

The greatest movement takes place in the flexures and in the transverse colon.

The diaphragm is the propelling force for the movement of the colic flexures: in the frontal plane, the diaphragmatic movement is greater on the side than in the center—the flexures move inferiorly and medially (approximately 3 cm in normal inhalations, up to 10 cm in maximum inhalation).

In the sagittal plane, the flexures move anteroinferiorly.

The transverse colon also moves inferiorly in the frontal plane, whereby the following applies: the fuller it is, the higher it lies.

Motility

Each part of the colon completes a transversal motion on its parietal attachment (Toldt fascia, mesocolon). This results in a mediolateral or superoinferior (for the transverse colon) concave distortion in the frontal plane.

In the same way, a rotation takes place around the longitudinal axis of the colon.

Physiology

In the colon, water and electrolytes are extracted from the chyme; the stool becomes thickened.

In addition, the feces can be stored in the sigmoid and rectum for several days.

Pathologies

Symptoms that Require Medical Clarification

- Signs of appendicitis on the right or left (diverticulitis)
- Bloody stools
- Change in bowel movements (longer than 3 weeks)

Appendicitis

Definition. Acute inflammation of the vermiform appendix with signs of an acute abdomen.

Causes. The cause is unknown.

Clinical.
- pain that begins in the epigastrium, sometimes colic-like, and moves into the right lower abdomen in the course of hours
- rectal–axillary temperature difference of more than 0.5 °C in temperatures of about 38 °C
- pain at the McBurney point and Lanz point
- rebound tenderness
- Blumberg sign (crossed rebound tenderness)
- Rovsing sign (retrograde compression of the colon)
- positive psoas test on the right
- Douglas pain

Ulcerative Colitis

Definition. Chronic inflammation of the large intestinal mucosa with ulcerations. The inflammation is limited to the mucosa and submucosa and spreads from the rectum proximally.

Causes. The cause is unknown. Possible causes include infections, and dietary, psychological, and immunological factors.

Familial aggregation occurs.

Clinical
- bloody/slimy diarrhea (guiding symptom)
- The disease erupts in episodes with symptom-free intervals.
- Depending on the severity of the disease, episodes can manifest with fever, abdominal spasms, and a definite feeling of sickness.

Irritable Bowel Syndrome

Definition. Functional intestinal disorder.

Causes. Psychological triggers.
Patients show the following characteristics:
- lowered pain threshold for stretch reflexes
- increased motor activity in the sigmoid colon
- changed transit time of food
- increased gas reflux in the stomach

Clinical
- sheep-dung or pencil-like stools
- mucus in the stool (without blood)
- diarrhea in the morning (the first stool is solid, the second soft, the third watery)
- variable abdominal pain, mostly on the left side
- food intolerances without proof of allergies
- vegetative symptoms (headache, insomnia, dysuria)
- overanxiousness
- dysmenorrhea
- carcinophobia
- improvement of symptoms during vacations

Diverticulitis

Definition. Inflammation of existing diverticula (pouches of mucosa and submucosa through the lamina propria) after pressure necrosis due to a coprolith.

Causes. Diverticula form as the result of large pressure differences in the sigmoid colon, with existing weakness of the connective tissue and chronic constipation.

Clinical
- "left-sided appendicitis"
- fever
- left-sided lower abdominal complaints with pressure pain and muscular defense

Colorectal Cancer

Definition. Adenocarcinoma of the colon.
After bronchial carcinoma, this is the second most common form of cancer in humans.

Causes
- adenomas (large intestinal polyps)
- high protein and fat consumption
- being overweight
- lack of dietary fiber
- familial aggregation
- total ulcerative colitis

Clinical
- bloody stools (occult or visible)
- changes in defecatory habits (longer than 3 weeks)
- signs of ileus
- weight loss
- fever
- anemia

Osteopathic Practice

Cardinal Symptoms

- Symptoms of appendicitis on the right or left
- Defecatory irregularities (change between constipation and diarrhea)
- Bloody stools

Typical Dysfunctions

- adhesions/fixations
- spasms with transit problem

Associated Structural Dysfunctions

- lumbosacral transition
- iliosacral joint

Atypical Symptoms

A list of symptoms follows that can be explained by means of osteopathic chains or result from the patient's history (for an explanation of osteopathic chains, see "Atypical Symptoms" in Chapter 5, page 39):
- feeling of heaviness or spasms in the abdomen
- flatulence
- prone position is uncomfortable

In contrast to other authors, Barral in addition lists the following organ-specific symptoms:
- coated tongue and bad breath
- fatigue in the late afternoon or fatigue with insomnia
- painful and light-sensitive eyes 3–4 hours after eating
- feeling of heaviness in the legs in the morning
- shallow breathing

- humeroscapular periarthritis
- constipation
- recurrent iliosacral joint pain
- recurrent blockages in the lumbosacral transition
- irritable bowel syndrome (irritable colon)

- inflammations
- tumors
- new scars

Osteopathic Tests and Treatment

Mobilization of the Cecum according to Barral

Starting Position
The patient is in the supine position, legs bent. The practitioner stands to the right of the patient.

Displaceability toward Medial

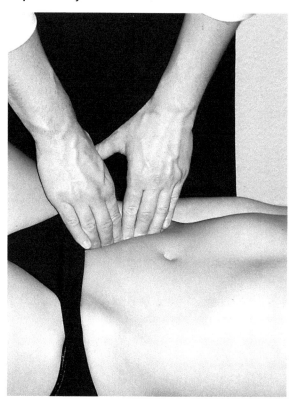

Fig. 13.4

Testing Sequence
Slide both hands on top of the iliacus and medial to the right ileum posteriorly. Displace the cecum medially and diagonally toward the left shoulder, to test the lateral attachments. Pay attention to soreness and abnormal tensions.

Treatment
Carry out treatment as described in the test. To improve mobility, you can apply a continuous pull, vibrations, or rebounds.

Displaceability toward Lateral

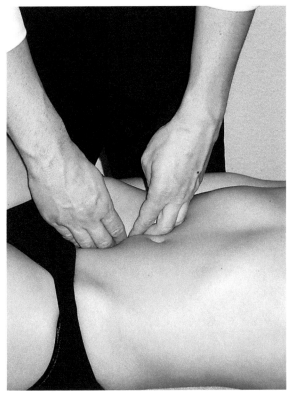

Fig. 13.5

Displaceability toward Cranial

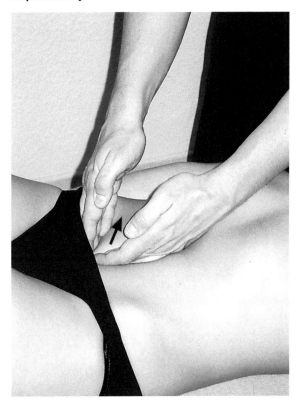

Fig. 13.6

Testing Sequence
Place both hands on the abdominal wall medial to the cecum and let them glide into the abdomen posteriorly. Displace the cecum laterally and diagonally toward the right hip. This action tests the medial attachments. Pay attention to soreness and abnormal tensions as well.

Treatment
Carry out treatment as described in the test. To improve mobility, you can apply a continuous pull, vibrations, or rebounds.

Testing Sequence
Place both hands on the abdominal wall caudal to the cecum and let them glide posteriorly. Displace the cecum cranially and slightly diagonally toward the right shoulder, to test the inferior attachments. Pay attention to soreness and abnormal tensions as well.

Variation
All three techniques can also be performed in other starting positions:
• lateral position facing left
• knee–elbow position

Combined Treatment of the Cecum with Leg Lever according to Barral

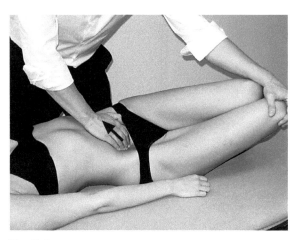

Fig. 13.7

Starting Position
The patient is in the supine position, legs bent. The practitioner stands on the patient's left side.

Procedure
The cranial hand glides into the depth on top of the iliacus and lateral to the cecum, pulling it in a cranial–medial direction toward the navel. The caudal hand holds the legs by the knees.

Treatment
While the cranial hand fixates the cecum, the caudal hand moves the legs rightward and downward onto the treatment table. You can hold this position or mobilize rhythmically.

This technique can also be applied to the ascending colon.

Mobilization of the Sigmoid Colon according to Barral

Starting Position
The patient is in the supine position, legs bent. The practitioner stands on the patient's left side.

Displaceability toward Medial

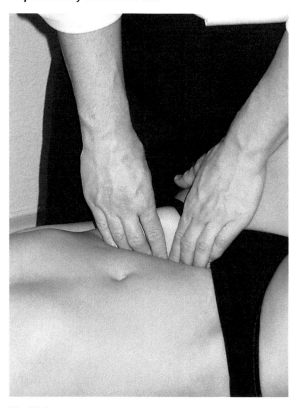

Fig. 13.8

Testing Sequence
Slide both hands on top of the iliacus and medial to the left ileum posteriorly. Displace the sigmoid medially and diagonally toward the navel, to test the lateral attachments. Pay attention to soreness and abnormal tensions.

Treatment
Carry out treatment as described in the test. To improve mobility, you can apply a continuous pull, vibrations, or rebounds.

Displaceability toward Lateral

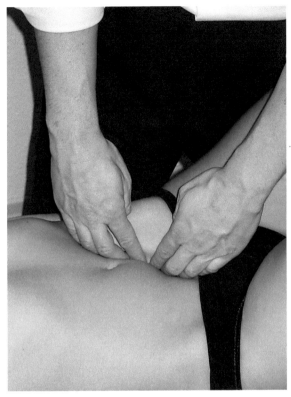

Fig. 13.9

Testing Sequence
Place both hands on the abdominal wall medial to the sigmoid and slide them posteriorly into the abdomen. Displace the sigmoid laterally and diagonally toward the left hip. This action tests the medial attachments. Pay attention to soreness and abnormal tensions.

Treatment
Carry out treatment as described in the test. To improve mobility, you can apply a continuous pull, vibrations, or rebounds.

Variation
All three techniques can also be performed in other starting positions:
- lateral position facing right
- knee–elbow position

Treatment of the Sigmoid Mesocolon

Starting Position
The patient is in the supine position, legs bent. The practitioner stands on the patient's left side.

Treatment of the Diagonally Running Section of the Mesocolon

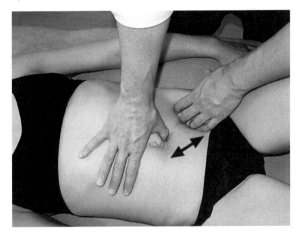

Fig. 13.10

Procedure
With the caudal hand, grasp a large section of the abdominal wall medial to the sigmoid in the region of the iliac fossa; place the cranial hand on the abdomen on the left, about 2–3 cm below the navel on a diagonal line connecting the navel and the hip.

Treatment
Slide both hands posteriorly. The sigmoid mesocolon is located between them. The stretch results from a simultaneous pull with both hands: the caudal hand pulls diagonally toward the left hip, the cranial hand diagonally toward the navel.

Treatment of the Craniocaudally Running Section of the Mesocolon

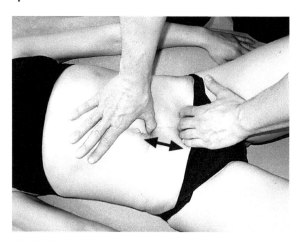

Fig. 13.11

Procedure

With the caudal hand, take hold of a large area of the abdominal wall left of the median line and medial to the sigmoid; place the cranial hand on the abdomen to the left of the median line, about 2–3 cm below the navel.

Treatment

Slide both hands posteriorly. The sigmoid mesocolon is located between them. The stretch results from a simultaneous pull with both hands: the caudal hand pulls straight down vertically, and the cranial hand pulls straight up vertically.

Combined Treatment of the Sigmoid with Leg Lever according to Barral

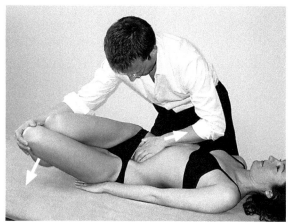

Fig. 13.12

Starting Position

The patient is in the supine position, legs bent. The practitioner stands on the patient's right side.

Procedure

The cranial hand glides into the depth on top of the iliacus on the lateral side of the sigmoid, pulling it in a cranial–medial direction toward the navel.

The caudal hand grasps the legs by the knees.

Treatment

While the cranial hand fixates the sigmoid, the caudal hand moves the legs rightward and downward onto the treatment table. You can hold this position or mobilize rhythmically.

You can also apply this technique to the descending colon.

Mobilization of the Ascending Colon according to Barral

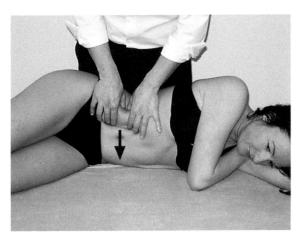

Fig. 13.13

Starting Position
The patient is in the lateral position facing left, legs bent. The practitioner stands behind the patient.

Procedure
With the thumbs of both hands reach into the abdomen posterior to the ascending colon. The fingers of both hands grip between the ascending colon and small intestinal loops. The ascending colon is now held by both hands.

Testing Sequence
Displace the colon medially in the direction of the navel. Then allow it to passively glide back. Pay attention to soreness and abnormal tensions.

Repeat this test in different locations on the ascending colon.

Treatment
You can also perform the described test as treatment. Mobilize the less mobile sections of the ascending colon rhythmically or hold the position at the end of the movement and apply small rebounds.

You can also apply this technique to the descending colon. Merely note that this section of the large intestine is located further posteriorly.

Lengthwise Stretch of the Ascending Colon according to Barral

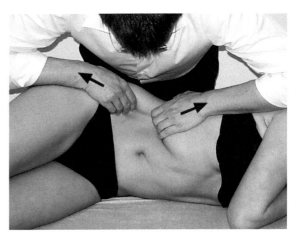

Fig. 13.14

Starting Position
The patient is in the lateral position facing left. The practitioner stands behind the patient.

Procedure
With the cranial hand, reach under the right costal arch and slide your fingers posterosuperiorly and laterally in the direction of the right colic flexure. Work the caudal hand into the abdomen at the height of the iliac crest onto the start section of the ascending colon—fixate the colon posteriorly.

Treatment
Guide the cranial hand posterosuperiorly and laterally while you mobilize the colon with the caudal hand caudally. This action results in a lengthwise stretch of the ascending colon.

This technique is also suitable for the descending colon—place the caudal hand on the inferior section of the descending colon.

Treatment of the Toldt Fascia according to Barral

Test and Treatment of the Colic Flexures according to Barral

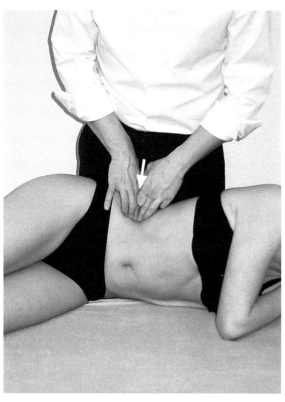

Fig. 13.15

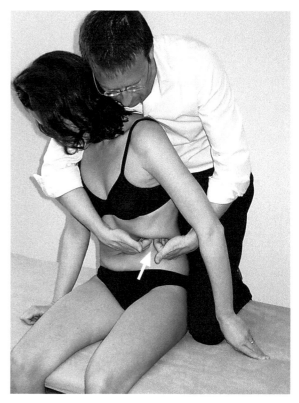

Fig. 13.16

Starting Position

The patient is in the lateral position facing left, legs slightly bent. The practitioner stands behind the patient.

Procedure

Sink the fingers of both hands deeply into the abdomen on the posterior side of the colon between the colon and the lateral abdominal wall.

Then, mobilize the fascia with constant pressure, vibrations, rebounds, or frictions.

This technique is also suitable for the descending colon.

Starting Position

The patient sits in a kyphotic position. The practitioner stands behind the patient.

Procedure

With your right arm, reach over the patient's right shoulder; with the left arm, reach under the patient's left armpit. Now place the fingers of both hands far lateral below the costal arch onto the abdominal wall; bring the patient into a kyphotic posture and slide deeply into the abdomen. For easier palpation of the flexure, bring the patient into ipsilateral lateral flexion and contralateral rotation.

The fingers advance posterosuperiorly and laterally. The flexure and the right or left phrenicocolic ligament can be evaluated for soreness and abnormal tonicity.

Treatment

To treat the phrenicocolic ligament, intermittently facilitate a contralateral lateral flexion and perform a stretch with the fingers by means of pressure superolaterally.

To treat the flexure, perform a stretch in a posterosuperior–lateral direction.

Rebounds, frictions, or vibrations are other potential techniques for this treatment.

Stretching Both Flexures Simultaneously according to Barral

Mobilization of the Flexures in the Sagittal Plane according to Barral

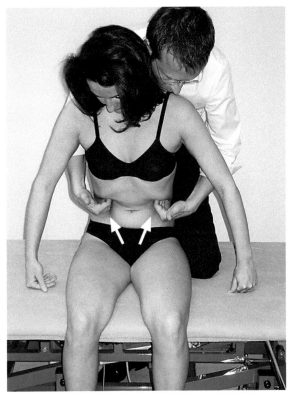

Fig. 13.17

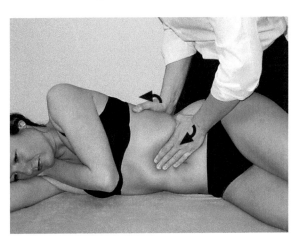

Fig. 13.18

Starting Position
The patient is seated. The practitioner stands behind the patient.

Procedure
With both hands, reach as far as possible under the costal arches in a posterosuperior–lateral direction toward the colic flexures and fixate them each with one hand.

Treatment
Bring the patient into a slight extension and pull toward you. In this way, the stretch in the flexures is increased laterally. Hold this position and perform an additional stretch with both hands in a posterosuperior–lateral direction.

This technique also has a mobilizing effect on the transverse colon.

Starting Position
The patient is in the lateral position. The practitioner stands behind the patient.

Procedure
Place the cranial hand posterior to the axillary line on the lower ribs and the caudal hand slightly anterior to the axillary line below the costal arch.

Treatment
With the caudal hand, mobilize the colon near the flexure anteromedially; with the cranial hand, bring the costal arch posterosuperiorly.

Cecum and Ascending Colon

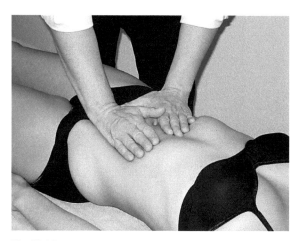

Fig. 13.19

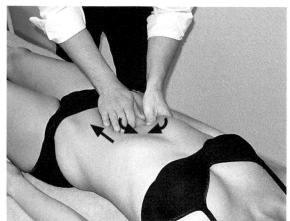

Fig. 13.20

Starting Position
The patient is in the supine position. The practitioner stands by the patient's right side.

Procedure
The fingers of the left hand lie on the ascending colon (thenar on the cecum); the fingers of the right hand rest on the descending colon (thenar on the sigmoid).

Testing Sequence
Detect the motility movement: during exhalation, the colon performs a clockwise rotation; the cecum and sigmoid also move superomedially. During inhalation, the movement runs in the opposite direction.

Evaluate the amplitude and direction of the inspiratory and expiratory movements as well as the rhythm of the movement as a whole. If a disturbance is present in one or both aspects of the motility movement, treat the patient.

Treatment
Motility is treated indirectly by following the unimpaired movement, remaining at the end-point of this movement for several cycles, and then following the impaired movement to the new end-point.

You can also try to increase the range of the free movement (induction), afterward checking whether the limited movement direction has improved.

Repeat this movement again and again until the motility has returned to normal in terms of rhythm, direction, and amplitude.

Starting Position
The patient is in the supine position. The practitioner stands on the patient's right side.

Procedure
Place the right hand on the cecum with the fingertips pointing in a medial–cranial direction toward the navel. The left hand grasps the flank as close as possible to the costal arch; the fingertips lie posterior. The ascending colon lies in your hand.

Treatment
During inhalation, pull with both hands caudally. The right hand rotates with the fingertips outward, while at the same time the left hand exerts pressure medially.

During exhalation, maintain the position reached. Repeat this procedure until you have reached the end of the fascial movement. During the next exhalation, release the pull.

Repeat the whole treatment four or five times.

Ascending Colon, Right Colic Flexure, Right Part of the Transverse Colon

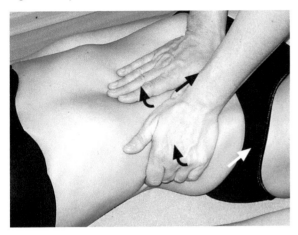

Fig. 13.21

Starting Position
The patient is in the supine position. The practitioner stands on the patient's left side.

Procedure
The left hand grasps the flank as close to the costal arch as possible; the fingertips lie posterior. The ascending colon lies in your hand. The right hand lies flat on the abdomen with the fingertips touching below the right costal arch. The fingers point toward the right shoulder.

Treatment
During inhalation, both hands simultaneously pull caudally and rotate clockwise. In this way, the right colic flexure is pulled in a caudal–left direction.

During exhalation, maintain the position reached. Repeat this treatment until you have reached the end of the fascial movement. During the next exhalation, release the pull.

Repeat the whole treatment four or five times.

Descending Colon and Sigmoid Colon

Starting Position
The patient is in the supine position. The practitioner stands on the patient's left side.

Procedure
The hand position and treatment are identical to the technique for the "Cecum and Ascending Colon." You merely have to transfer it to the other side.

Left Part of the Transverse Colon, Left Colic Flexure, Descending Colon

Starting Position
The patient is in the supine position. The practitioner stands on the patient's right side.

Procedure
The hand position is identical to the technique for the "Ascending Colon, Right Colic Flexure, Right Part of the Transverse Colon." You merely have to transfer it to the other side.

Treatment
During inhalation, pull with both hands caudally. The right hand in addition rotates in the counterclockwise direction and the left hand in the clockwise direction. In this way, the left flexure is mobilized caudally.

During exhalation, maintain the position reached. Repeat this procedure until you have reached the end of the fascial movement. During the next exhalation, release the pull.

Repeat the whole treatment three or four times.

Circulatory Treatment according to Kuchera

Arterial Stimulation

- stimulation of the superior and inferior mesenteric arteries by working on the spinal column
- diaphragm techniques

Venous Stimulation

- liver pump
- stretching the hepatoduodenal ligament
- diaphragm techniques

Lymphatic Stimulation

- lymph drainage on thorax and abdomen
- diaphragm techniques

Vegetative Harmonization

Sympathetic nervous system:
Stimulation of the sympathetic trunk T10–L2 by:
- rib raising
- inhibiting the paravertebral muscles
- vibrations
- manipulations
- Maitland technique
- stimulation of the superior and inferior mesenteric ganglia
- diaphragm techniques

Parasympathetic nervous system:
Stimulation of the vagus nerve by:
- craniosacral therapy
- laryngeal techniques
- thoracic techniques (recoil)
- diaphragm techniques

Stimulation of segments S2–S4 by:
- iliosacral joint techniques
- ischiorectal fossa technique
- treatment of the pelvic floor

Reflex Point Treatment according to Chapman

Location for the Mesoappendix

Anterior. At the upper edge of rib 12, near the tip of the rib—only on the right!

Posterior. Medial border of the eleventh intercostal space.

Location for the Rectum

Anterior. From the lesser trochanter downward (on both sides).

Posterior. On the sacrum near the ilium at the lower end of the iliosacral joint (on both sides).

Location for the Colon

Anterior. A 2.5- to 5-cm wide zone from the greater trochanter to approximately 3 cm above the patella on the frontolateral thigh (on both sides).

Right side. Diagnostically, the first one-fifth from cranial represents the cecum, the next three-fifths the ascending colon, and the caudal one-fifth the transverse colon.

Left side. The caudal one-fifth represents the transverse colon, the next three-fifths cranially the descending colon, and the highest one-fifth the sigmoid colon.

Posterior. A triangular area that stretches between the tip of the transverse process of L2–L4 and the iliac crest (on both sides).

Treatment Principle

Make contact with the reflex point. For this purpose, very gently place a finger on the point and exert only light pressure. Reflex points are often very sensitive, and it is therefore important to proceed with caution.

The finger remains on the point and treatment is by gentle rotations.

The anterior points are treated first, then the posterior points. Continue with the treatment until you have normalized the soreness or consistency of the point.

To conclude, check the anterior points once more. If you fail to notice any change, it is possible that the organ pathology is too great to be influenced quickly via the reflex points, or there are other dysfunctions present that must be treated first.

Recommendations for the Patient

- Eat only light meals in the evening.
- Consume foods rich in dietary fiber.
- Stimulate the liver and pancreas with olive oil, lemon, or herbs.

14 The Kidneys

Anatomy

General Facts

Size: 12 cm long, 7 cm wide, and 3 cm thick.

Location

Posterior
Left kidney:
Upper pole: T11
Renal pelvis: L1
Lower pole: L3

The **right kidney** is located approximately 1–1.5 cm lower than the left kidney.

Anterior
Left kidney:
Upper pole: rib 9
Lower pole: 1–2 cm above the navel
Right kidney:
Upper pole: rib 9
Lower pole: level of the navel

The axis of the kidney runs slightly diagonally from cranial–medial to caudal–lateral.

Renal Fascia

This consists of an anterior leaf and a posterior leaf. Both leaves merge superior and lateral to the kidneys. This "fascial sac" is open on the bottom.

The fascias of both kidneys merge at the level T12–L1 in front of the spinal column.

Retrorenal lamina:
This covers quadratus lumborum and psoas major and is fixed anteriorly and laterally to the spinal column (medial to the psoas and diaphragm).

Prerenal lamina:
This lies next to the peritoneum and Toldt fascia. On the left side, it is associated with this fascia in a larger area. It covers the kidney, hilum, and the large prevertebral vessels.

Both laminae surround the adrenal glands, merge superiorly, and are attached to the diaphragm.

Inside the fascial layers and surrounding the kidney, we find fat (fat capsule). This exists from about age 10 on.

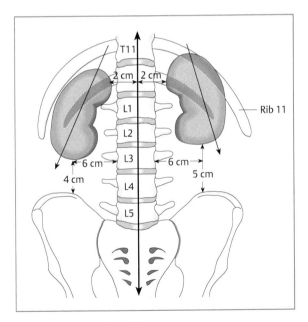

Fig. 14.1 Location of the kidneys.

Topographic Relationships

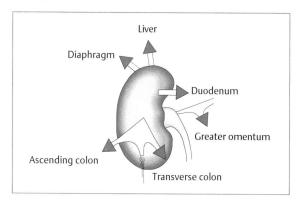

Fig. 14.2 Connections of the right kidney.

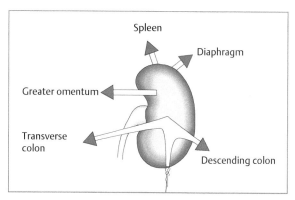

Fig. 14.3 Connections of the left kidney.

Posterior
- diaphragm and psoas arcade
- pleura (indirectly in the area of the costodiaphragmatic recess up to the level of L1)
- rib 12, on the left also rib 11
- psoas major and its fascia
- quadratus lumborum and transversus abdominis
- subcostal, iliohypogastric, ilioinguinal nerves
- Grynfeltt triangle

Anterior
Right kidney:
- liver
- hepatoduodenal ligament
- right colic flexure
- transverse mesocolon
- duodenum, descending part
- ascending colon

Left kidney:
- spleen
- stomach
- pancreas
- duodenojejunal flexure
- jejunum
- left colic flexure (stronger fixation than on the right)

The adrenal glands lie superior to both kidneys.

Attachments/Suspensions

- turgor
- pressure of other organs and tonicity of the abdominal muscles
- fat capsule
- hilar vessels and ureter (braking function)
- thoracic suction effect and tonicity of the abdominal muscles during respiration

Circulation

Arterial

Renal artery (originates in the aorta, roughly 1 cm below the superior mesenteric artery; the left one is shorter than the right one).

Venous

Renal vein (left vein is longer than the right one, ends in the inferior vena cava).

Lymph Drainage

- lumbar nodes
- lumbar trunk
- thoracic duct

Innervation

- sympathetic nervous system from T10 to L1 via the lesser and lowest splanchnic nerves and the lumbar splanchnic nerves 1 and 2 to the celiac plexus, aorticorenal ganglion, renal plexus, and posterior renal ganglion
- vagus nerves (via the celiac plexus)
- sacral parasympathetic part (S2–S4) via the superior hypogastric plexus to the renal plexus

Organ Clock

Maximal time: 5–7 p.m.
Minimal time: 5–7 a.m.

Organ–Tooth Interrelationship

For basic information, see page 34.

- Second incisor in the lower jaw on both sides
- First incisor in the upper jaw on both sides

Movement Physiology according to Barral

Three factors determine the movement of the kidneys:
1. The renal fascia is open toward the bottom and medially.
2. The hilum vessels pull on the kidney.
3. The psoas is a slide rail.

Mobility

The engine of this movement is the diaphragm. During inhalation (20000/day, 600m/day), the kidney moves 3–4cm caudally.

The upper pole is pressed forward during inhalation (psoas slide rail). In addition, the kidney moves in a caudal–lateral direction and rotates outward.

Motility

During inhalation, we feel a movement from medial–cranial to lateral–caudal in connection with an outward rotation ("windshield wiper"). During exhalation, the kidney completes the opposite movement.

Physiology

Functions of the Kidney

- regulation of the fluids and electrolytes
- regulation of the acid–base balance
- excretion of substances through the urine (urea, creatinine, uric acid, etc.)
- excretion of foreign substances (medications)
- regulation of blood pressure (renin–angiotensin–aldosterone system)
- hormone production (erythropoietin, renin, calcitriol, prostaglandins)
- degradation of peptide hormones

Pathologies

Symptoms that Require Medical Clarification

> - Pain elicited by percussion in the kidney area
> - Hematuria

Nephrolithiasis

Definition. Urinary stones in the kidney and excretory urinary tracts.

Causes. Excessive amounts of stone-forming substances in the urine.

Risk factors include:
- lack of physical movement
- insufficient fluid supply
- familial predisposition
- medications (calcium, vitamin C and D therapy)
- gout
- diabetes mellitus
- kidney disorders
- hyperparathyroidism

Clinical. Asymptomatic if the calculi do not constrict the urinary tracts.

Obstructing stone causes:
- colic with hematuria
- nausea
- vomiting
- abdominal pain
- flank pain
- pain radiating into the genitals and inside of the thighs

Acute Pyelonephritis

Definition. Infection of the upper urinary tract caused by pathogenic organisms.

Causes. Highly virulent organisms coinciding with a weakened state of defense.

Precipitating factors include:
- stricture of the urinary tract
- vesicoureteral reflux
- neurogenic disturbance of bladder voiding
- calculi
- diabetes mellitus
- immunosuppressive therapy

Clinical
- pain elicited by percussion in the kidney area
- flank pain
- headache
- sweating
- nausea
- vomiting
- fever >38.5 °C

Nephrotic Syndrome

Definition. Complex of symptoms, consisting of:
- proteinuria
- hypoproteinemia
- dysproteinemia
- hyperlipoproteinemia
- edemas

Causes. We find primary or secondary preexisting glomerular disorders, e.g.:
- poststreptococcal glomerulonephritis
- rapidly progressive glomerulonephritis
- systemic disorders, e.g., lupus erythematosus

Clinical
- microhematuria
- edemas
- hypertonicity

Renal Cell Carcinoma

Definition. Most common form of malignant tumor in the kidney, in most cases originating in the tubular cells.

Causes. Degeneration of proximal tubular cells.

Clinical
- hematuria
- elevated ESR
- palpable abdominal mass
- hypertonicity
- weight loss
- anemia
- intermittent fever
- asymptomatic in the early stages

Osteopathic Practice

Cardinal Symptoms

> - Pain elicited by percussion in the kidney area
> - Hematuria

Typical Dysfunctions

- ptosis
- adhesions/fixations

Theory of Kidney Ptosis according to Barral

Causes
- ptosis up to the lesser pelvis is congenital
- asthenic body
- trauma (fall on the coccyx, vibrations)
- rapid and extensive weight loss
- depression
- turgor effect decreases with increasing age
- ptosis after childbirth
- suction from below and pressure from above during delivery
- loose ligaments

Ptosis of the Right Kidney

"Digestive kidney." This name stems from the fact that the digestive tract has such a strong influence on the right kidney. See also "Notes for Clinical Application," page 143.

The liver and ascending colon are the main factors affecting the kidney.

Ptosis of the right kidney is more common than ptosis of the left kidney because:
- the large liver presses down more strongly
- the Toldt fascia is weaker on the right side
- the left colic flexure fixates more strongly
- the scoliosis in the lumbar spinal column (LSC) brings the right kidney to anterior, which increases the pressure from the liver

Ptosis of the Left Kidney

Genital kidney. This name stems from the fact that the ovarian/testicular vein has such a strong influence on the left kidney. See also "Notes for Clinical Application," page 143.

Symptoms include:
- varicocele
- left-sided dysmenorrhea
- loss of libido
- impotence

The left ovarian/testicular vein runs into the left renal vein, on the right side directly into the inferior vena cava.

Degree of Ptosis

First degree
- ptosis runs caudally
- subcostal nerve is irritated

Symptoms include:
- diffuse pain in the area of the lower ribs
- sharp pain in the area of the lower ribs, radiating in the direction of the navel and disturbed breathing

Second degree
- The kidney shifts in a caudal–lateral direction, the outward rotation is intensified, and the lower pole moves to anterior (psoas as the slide rail).
- The genitofemoral, lateral femoral cutaneous, ilioinguinal, and iliohypogastric nerves are irritated.

Symptoms include: corresponding to the area innervated by the irritated nerves, patients can experience pain in the area of the groin, the lateral hip region and the lateral thigh, medial thigh, or in the area of the genitals.

Third degree
- The lower pole droops in a caudal–medial direction with an inward rotation (caused by the pull of the vessels and the ureter).

- The inward rotation is tolerated better than the outward rotation. The psoas no longer serves as a slide rail.
- The femoral nerve is irritated.

Symptom: knee pain (increased by flexion).

Associated Structural Dysfunctions

- T11–T12 and costovertebral joints of T10–B1
- L1–L2 (due to neurovegetative reflexes)
- coccyx
- dysfunctions of the ileum

Atypical Symptoms

In contrast to other authors, Barral additionally lists the following organ-specific symptoms (for an explanation of osteopathic chains, see "Atypical Symptoms" in Chapter 5, page 39):
- polyuria with great thirst in the early morning or during the night
- abdominal discomfort with dyspnea
- pain below the diaphragm or in the lesser pelvis
- LSC pain disappears shortly after getting up
- LSC pain during the day due to "stresses" such as coughing, sneezing, prolonged sitting or standing, tight belts
- gingivitis, aphthosis, stomatitis
- dry skin
- patient is flexed, holds the stomach or the lower posterior ribs
- when sneezing or coughing, patient flexes the hip on the affected side, to compensate for the increased pressure

Indications for Osteopathic Treatment

- ptosis
- adhesions/fixations

Contraindications for Osteopathic Treatment

- acute inflammation
- hematuria
- carcinoma
- cystic kidney

Notes for Clinical Application

As an organ, the kidney functions as the body's filter. To perform this task, the kidney has an enormous compensatory capability: 75% of its filtration capacity can fail, without any effect on the body. We know that a person can live well with only one kidney, but even the remaining single kidney must fail at more than 50% before we speak of kidney insufficiency. This immense compensatory capability means that the kidney can compensate well for a diversity of disturbing factors. This fact also holds true for osteopathic dysfunctions. In the author's opinion, it is rare to find the kidney as the primary cause of symptoms; it is much more likely that it is reacting to another organ, which can certainly also trigger parietal symptoms, but the kidney itself will not be impaired in its function.

Let us look at an example to illustrate this point: parietal symptoms that are likely to arise with an osteopathic dysfunction of the kidney can be explained by the three nerves of the lumbar plexus, which are found posterior to the kidney on the psoas major. These are the subcostal, iliohypogastric, and ilioinguinal nerves. The pain that is characteristic of a renal colic can be interpreted as irritations of these nerves due to a congested kidney. The same holds true for osteopathic dysfunctions. Whether it is a disturbance in the slide bearing or a circulatory impairment in the osteopathic sense that is disturbing the kidney, the three lumbar plexus nerves are irritated, resulting in pain e.g., in the groin or in the lateral trochanter area. It is easy to confuse this with a coxarthrosis or a trochanteric bursitis. In the osteopathic context, we also like to speak of a congested kidney that is pressing on the nerves. Here, it is important to point out specifically that we are not dealing with an engorged kidney. In this osteopathic dysfunction, the function of the kidney is not impaired!

What Factors Can Trigger Such a Dysfunction?

The right kidney is also known as the digestive kidney because the various organs of the digestive system can irritate this kidney. The first organ to mention here is the liver, which lies on top of the right kidney. If the liver is congested, it transmits increased pressure posteriorly to the kidney, which subsequently develops a disturbance in the slide bearing.

The transition from the superior part to the descending part of the duodenum is located at the renal pelvis. This section of the duodenum is frequently affected by osteopathic dysfunctions as the result of ulcers that form most commonly in the superior part. This condition then has a secondary detrimental effect on the kidney and its circulation.

The ascending colon likewise has contact with the kidney at its lower pole.

The ureter is crossed by the root of the mesentery near the ileocecal valve; as a result, a ptosis of the small intestine can have a constricting effect on the ureter, which in turn can result in an osteopathic congestion of the kidney.

The left kidney is also known as the genital kidney, which points to the fact that the primary sexual organs can affect this kidney. The reason for this is that the ovarian or testicular vein on the left side runs into the renal vein, while it drains its blood on the right side into the inferior vena cava. An increased blood flow into the renal vein can hence lead to signs of congestion in the kidney on the left side.

On the other hand, however, a section of the colon has an effect on the left kidney that should not be underestimated. The sigmoid colon has a mesentery that crosses both the ureter and the ovarian and testicular veins. Constipation, diverticulitis, and irritable bowel syndrome are three common disorders that affect the sigmoid and therefore in turn cause secondary dysfunction in the kidney.

In all cases mentioned here, the kidney responds to the dysfunction of another organ. On the right side, it is the organs of the digestive tract that affect the kidney; on the left side, it is the sexual organs and the large intestine. In functional terms, however, its great compensatory capacity protects it from being impaired. Nevertheless, parietal symptoms can still occur, which could lead us to focus treatment on the kidney and regard it as the primary cause. According to the author's experience, the other organs mentioned above are more likely to be the cause of the complaints, so we should treat these first. Afterward check to see whether dysfunction of the kidney is still present.

Osteopathic Tests and Treatment

The mobility of the kidney is more important than its position.

Palpation of the Kidney according to Barral

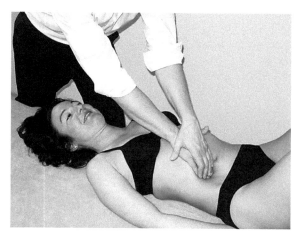

Fig. 14.4

Starting Position
The patient is in the supine position, legs bent. The practitioner stands by the patient's head on the contralateral side.

Procedure for the Right Kidney

Make contact with the abdominal wall on the right side, roughly at the level of the ileocecal valve. Carefully pushing the loops of the small intestine aside, slide cranially along the medial edge of the ascending colon.

Roughly at the height of the navel, you can palpate the kidney as a smooth solid mass (like a soap).

Normally, it is the anterior surface that is palpable, as well as the inferior pole in the case of a ptosis or in slim people.

Procedure for the Left Kidney

Make contact with the abdominal wall on the left side above the sigmoid in the caudal quarter of a line from the navel to the anterosuperior iliac spine (ASIS). Carefully pushing the loops of the small intestine aside, slide cranially along the medial edge of the descending colon.

The anterior surface or inferior pole is palpable roughly 1 cm above the navel.

You can also carry out either of these palpations with the patient in the seated position.

Variation for the Right Kidney

Starting Position

The patient is in the supine position, legs bent. The practitioner stands next to the patient on the side to be examined.

Procedure

With the thumb of the left hand, carefully work your way from lateral into the abdomen at the level of the navel. The thumb then lies on the medial edge of the ascending colon. The right hand pushes the mass of intestines toward the palpating thumb to cause a fascial release in the area of palpation.

The kidney is palpable as a solid mass.

Variation for the Left Kidney

Starting Position

The patient is in the supine position, legs bent. The practitioner stands next to the patient on the side to be examined.

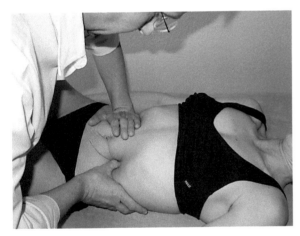

Fig. 14.5

Procedure

With the thumb of the right hand, carefully work your way from lateral into the abdomen roughly 1 cm above the navel. The thumb then lies on the medial edge of the descending colon. The left hand pushes the mass of intestines toward the palpating thumb to cause a fascial release in the area of palpation.

The kidney is palpable as a solid mass.

Mobilization of the Kidney

In the Supine Position according to Barral

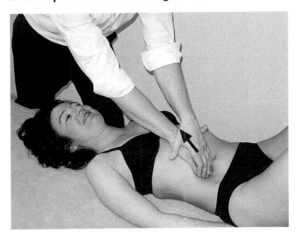

Fig. 14.6

Starting Position

The patient is in the supine position, legs bent. The practitioner stands by the patient's head on the contralateral side.

Procedure

Palpate the kidney as described on page 144.

Treatment

During the exhalation, mobilize the kidney along its axis of movement in a cranial–medial direction. During inhalation, hold the position reached.

Repeat this treatment several times.

In the Seated Position according to Barral

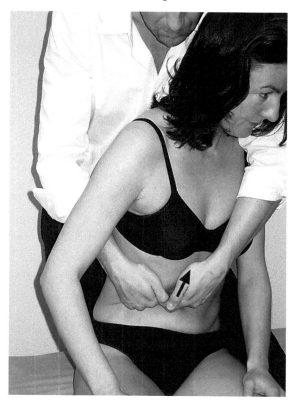

Fig. 14.7

Starting Position
The patient sits in kyphotic position. The practitioner stands behind the patient.

Procedure
Stand behind the patient and make contact with the kidney as described above.

Treatment
During the exhalation, mobilize the kidney along its axis of movement in a cranial–medial direction. During inhalation, hold the position reached.

Repeat this treatment several times.

In addition, you can facilitate a contralateral rotation of the torso. This action brings the kidney to the front, making it easier to palpate and therefore also easier to mobilize.

With the Aid of the Psoas Major according to Barral

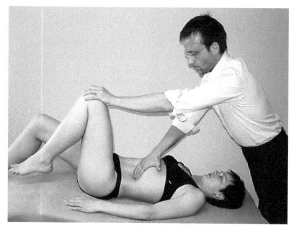

Fig. 14.8

Starting Position
The patient is in the supine position, legs bent, head down. The practitioner stands at the head of the table.

Procedure
Find the inferior pole of the kidney. Flex the patient's ipsilateral hip and hold the leg, while fixating the kidney with the palpating hand in a cranial–medial direction.

Treatment
During exhalation, guide the leg into extension, stretch the psoas, and mobilize the kidney by switching the fixed and mobile points.

You can combine this extension with an abduction or adduction of the hip to achieve an additional mobilizing aspect.

With Involvement of the Psoas Major and Post-Isometric Relaxation according to Barral

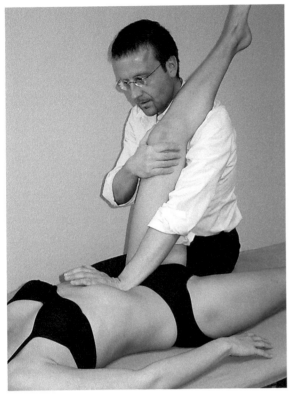

Fig. 14.9

Starting Position
The patient is in the supine position, legs bent. The practitioner stands next to the patient on the side to be examined.

Procedure
Place the patient's leg of the side to be treated onto your shoulder. With one hand, make contact with the inferior pole of the kidney. With the other hand, grasp the thigh of the leg on your shoulder from anterior. This hip bend creates tension in the psoas. During the exhalation, mobilize the kidney in a cranial–medial direction.

In addition, you can request isometric contractions of the psoas. During the exhalation and relaxation phase, finally mobilize the kidney.

By approximating the psoas, you create a slide rail for the kidney posterocranially.

Treatment of Grynfeltt Triangle according to Barral

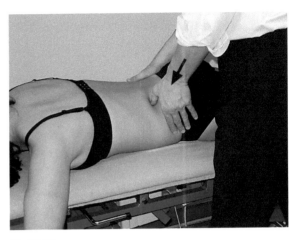

Fig. 14.10

Starting Position
The patient is in the prone position, legs stretched out. The practitioner stands next to the patient.

Procedure
Using one or two fingers, one hand makes contact with rib 12 posteriorly. Palpate it caudally in the direction of the iliac crest. Medial to the internal oblique muscle of the abdomen, you will find a muscle compartment formed by the tendon sheet of transversus abdominis. The kidney is located anterior to this compartment and should be treated via the Grynfeltt triangle. Leave your fingers there and push anterosuperiorly to mobilize the kidney.

Variation
You can place the other hand anteriorly onto the kidney and support the mobilization.

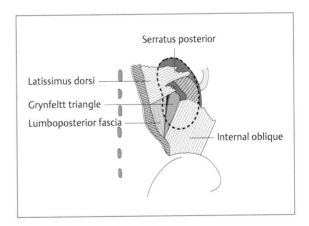

Fig. 14.11 Grynfeltt triangle.

Test and Treatment of Kidney Motility according to Barral

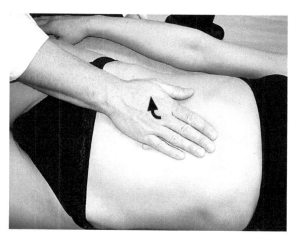

Fig. 14.12

Fascial Treatment according to Finet and Williame

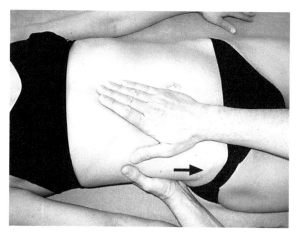

Fig. 14.13

Starting Position

The patient is in the supine position, legs stretched out. The practitioner stands next to the patient on the side to be examined.

Procedure

Place your hand with light pressure on the abdomen above the kidney, medial to the sigmoid or cecum. The forearm of the palpating hand lies on the abdomen.

Testing Sequence

Detect the motility motion and evaluate the amplitude and direction of the inspiratory and expiratory movements as well as the rhythm of the movement as a whole. If a disturbance is present in one or both aspects of the motility movement, treat the patient.

Treatment

Motility is treated indirectly by following the unimpaired movement, remaining at the end-point of this movement for several cycles, and then following the impaired movement to the new end-point.

You can also try to increase the range of the free movement (induction), afterward checking whether the limited movement direction has improved.

Repeat this movement again and again until the motility has returned to normal in terms of rhythm, direction, and amplitude.

Starting Position

The patient is in the supine position, legs stretched out. The practitioner stands next to the patient.

Procedure

Place your anterior hand on the abdomen on top of the projection of the kidney—the fingers pointing in a cranial–medial direction. The posterior hand rests at a corresponding height on the posterior wall of the torso—the fingertips pointing toward the spinal column. With the anterior hand, apply pressure posteriorly until you reach the fascial plane.

Treatment

During inhalation, both hands simultaneously pull caudally. During exhalation, hold the position reached. Repeat this procedure until you have reached the end of the fascial movement. Release the pull with the next exhalation.

Repeat the whole treatment four or five times.

Circulatory Treatment according to Kuchera

Arterial Stimulation

Diaphragm techniques.

Venous Stimulation

* liver pump
* diaphragm techniques

Lymphatic Stimulation

* lymph drainage on thorax and abdomen
* diaphragm techniques

Vegetative Harmonization   •

Sympathetic nervous system:
Stimulation of the sympathetic trunk T10–L1 by:
- rib raising
- inhibiting the paravertebral muscles
- vibrations
- manipulations
- Maitland technique
- stimulating the aorticorenal ganglion (technique as for the superior mesenteric ganglion)
- diaphragm techniques

Parasympathetic nervous system:
Stimulation of the vagus nerve by:
- craniosacral therapy
- laryngeal techniques
- thoracic techniques (recoil)
- diaphragm techniques

Stimulation of segments S2–S4 by:
- iliosacral joint techniques
- ischiorectal fossa technique
- pelvic floor

Reflex Point Treatment according to Chapman

Location

Anterior. Approximately 2.5 cm to both sides of the median line and approximately 2.5 cm cranial to the navel.

Posterior. Between the two transverse processes of T12 and L1, halfway between the spinous process and the tip of the transverse process (on both sides).

Treatment Principle

Make contact with the reflex point. For this purpose, very gently place a finger on the point and press only lightly. Reflex points are often very sensitive, so it is important to proceed with caution.

The finger remains on the point and treatment is by gentle rotations.

The anterior points are treated first, then the posterior points. Continue with the treatment until you have normalized the sensitivity or consistency of the point.

To conclude, check the anterior points once more. If you fail to notice any change, it is possible that the organ pathology is too great to be influenced quickly via the reflex points, or other dysfunctions are present that must be treated first.

Recommendations for the Patient

- Head-down position on an empty stomach with self-mobilization.
- In patients with lax fixations, strong coughing or sneezing can promote a ptosis.
- Ensure a sufficient supply of fluids.
- Diluted lemon juice increases the effectiveness of kidney manipulations.

15 The Urinary Bladder

Anatomy

▦ Anatomy of the Urinary Bladder

General Facts

The bladder's normal capacity lies at 500 mL, but strong urinary urgency occurs already with 300 mL.

In patients with voiding dysfunctions after surgery, up to 2000 mL can collect.

Location

The urinary bladder is located in the lesser pelvis behind the symphysis. An empty bladder does not extend with its superior pole beyond the symphysis; a full bladder can be palpated up to 3 cm above the symphysis.

Topographic Relationships

Female Pelvis

Superior
* peritoneum
* small intestinal loops
* uterus (depending on location)

Anterior
* pubis
* peritoneum
* when bladder is full: anterior abdominal wall

Inferior
* uterine cervix
* vagina
* urethra
* pelvic floor (levator ani)
* obturator internus

Posterior
* uterine cervix and isthmus
* vagina
* ureter

Lateral. Peritoneum, runs into the broad ligament of the uterus.

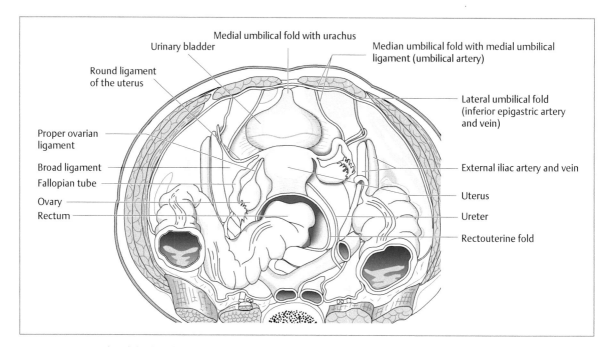

Fig. 15.1 Topography of the female lesser pelvis.

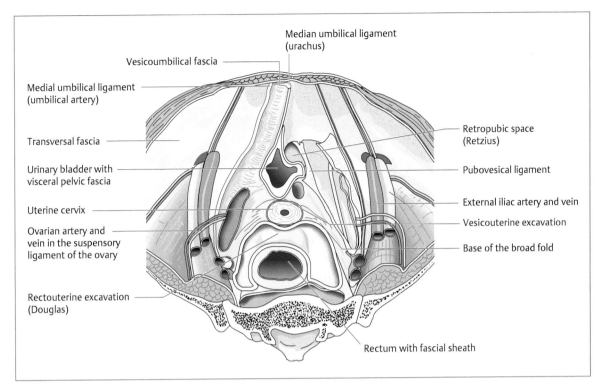

Fig. 15.2 Fascial attachments of the organs in the lesser pelvis.

Median umbilical ligament (urachus)

Vesicoumbilical fascia

Medial umbilical ligament (umbilical artery)

Transversal fascia

Urinary bladder with visceral pelvic fascia

Uterine cervix

Ovarian artery and vein in the suspensory ligament of the ovary

Rectouterine excavation (Douglas)

Retropubic space (Retzius)

Pubovesical ligament

External iliac artery and vein

Vesicouterine excavation

Base of the broad fold

Rectum with fascial sheath

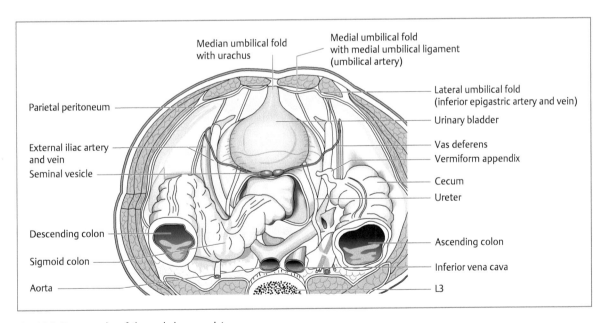

Fig. 15.3 Topography of the male lesser pelvis.

Median umbilical fold with urachus

Medial umbilical fold with medial umbilical ligament (umbilical artery)

Parietal peritoneum

External iliac artery and vein

Seminal vesicle

Descending colon

Sigmoid colon

Aorta

Lateral umbilical fold (inferior epigastric artery and vein)

Urinary bladder

Vas deferens

Vermiform appendix

Cecum

Ureter

Ascending colon

Inferior vena cava

L3

Male Pelvis

Superior
- peritoneum
- intestinal loops

Anterior
- pubis
- peritoneum
- when bladder is full: anterior abdominal wall

Inferior. Prostate gland.

Posterior
- vas deferens
- seminal vesicle
- rectum
- ureter
- peritoneum
- small intestinal loops

Lateral
- peritoneum
- levator ani
- obturator internus

Retropubic space (Retzius space):
Located between the pubic bone/abdominal wall and the urinary bladder, bordered caudally by the pubovesical ligament and medially by the median umbilical ligament.

Attachments/Suspensions

- peritoneum (anterior, lateral, and in men also posterior attachment)
- median umbilical ligament (with urachus)
- medial umbilical ligament (obliterated umbilical artery)
- pubovesical ligament (with muscle fibers from the bladder), corresponds to the puboprostatic ligament
- connective tissue of the lesser pelvis

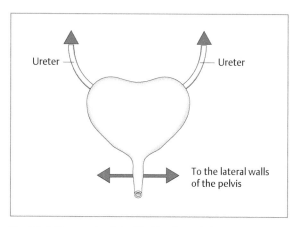

Fig. 15.4 Ligaments of the bladder, frontal view.

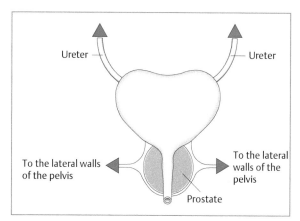

Fig. 15.6 Ligaments of the bladder, side view, in the male body.

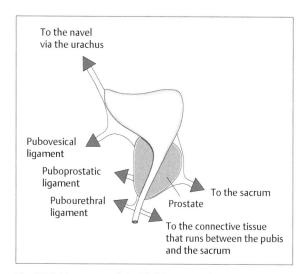

Fig. 15.5 Ligaments of the bladder, sagittal view.

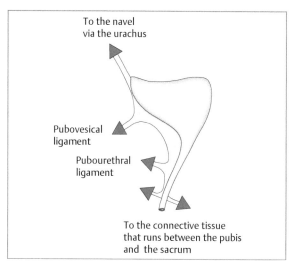

Fig. 15.7 Ligaments of the bladder, in the male body (view from the front).

Circulation

Arterial

Branches of the internal iliac artery, e.g.:
- inferior vesical artery
- internal pudendal artery
- obturator artery

Venous

- vesical venous plexus (anastomoses to the prostatic and vaginal venous plexus)
- internal iliac vein

Lymph Drainage

Internal and external iliac nodes.

Innervation

- sympathetic nervous system from L1 to L2 via the intermesenteric plexus and hypogastric nerves to the inferior hypogastric plexus and vesical plexus
- sacral parasympathetic nervous system (S2–S4) via the inferior hypogastric plexus and vesical plexus

Organ Clock

Maximal time: 3–5 p.m.
Minimal time: 3–5 a.m.

Organ–Tooth Interrelationship

For basic information, see page 34.

- First incisor in the lower jaw on both sides
- Second incisor in the upper jaw on both sides

■ Anatomy of the Ureter

General Facts

The ureter is 25–30 cm long and approximately 5 mm thick.

There are three physiologic bottlenecks where kidney stones are most likely to get impacted:
1. Transition from the renal pelvis into the ureter.
2. Sharp bend by the common/external iliac artery.
3. Passage into the urinary bladder (= narrowest point).

Location

The ureter runs caudal on top of the psoas major, passes across the bifurcation of the common iliac artery (left) or the external iliac artery (right) as it enters the lesser pelvis, and then descends further caudally along the lateral wall of the pelvis near the peritoneum.

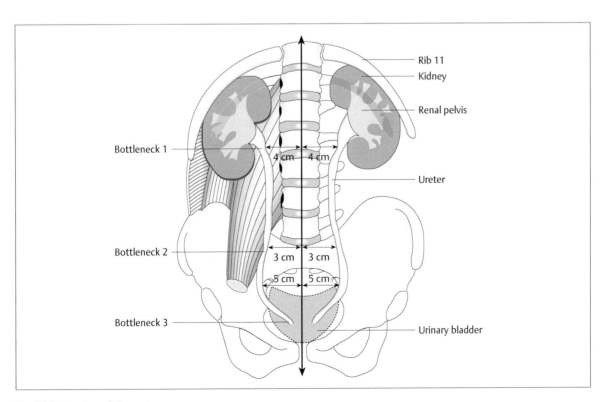

Fig. 15.8 Location of the ureter.

Continued Path in the Male Body

Roughly at the level of the ischiadic spine, it changes its course medially and anteriorly in the direction of the urinary bladder. Slightly above the seminal vesicle, it reaches the posterior lateral wall of the bladder, where it is crossed by the vas deferens. Here, the vas deferens lies closer to the peritoneum than the ureter. Continuing on, the ureter crosses the bladder diagonally from posterolateral to anteromedial.

Continued Path in the Female Body

Roughly at the level of the ischiadic spine, it changes its course medially and anteriorly in the direction of the urinary bladder. It initially lies in the base of the broad ligament of the uterus, and then it is crossed by the uterine artery. In its continued path, it proceeds at a distance of about 1–2 cm away from the supravaginal part of the uterine cervix. Right in front of the urinary bladder, it lies on top of the anterior and lateral vaginal vault. Entry into the urinary bladder takes place diagonally, as in the male body.

Topographic Relationships

See "Location"; in addition:
- peritoneum
- psoas fascia
- genitofemoral nerve
- inferior vena cava (right)
- duodenum (right)
- testicular/ovarian vessel
- right colic artery
- ileocolic artery
- inferior mesenteric artery or left colic artery
- root of the mesentery
- root of the sigmoid mesocolon

Attachments/Suspensions

- adipose capsule of the kidney
- peritoneum
- retro- and extraperitoneal connective tissue

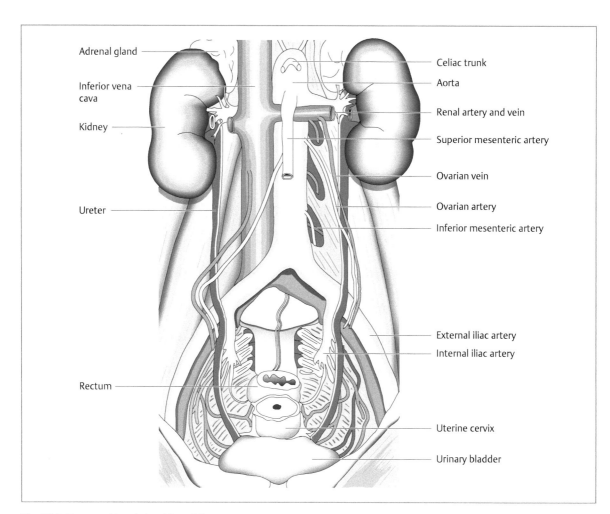

Fig. 15.9 Topographic relationships of the ureter.

Circulation

Arterial

The arterial supply is provided by branches of the arteries in its vicinity:
- renal artery
- abdominal aorta
- testicular/ovarian artery
- common iliac artery
- internal iliac artery
- inferior vesical artery
- uterine artery

Venous

- testicular/ovarian vein
- internal iliac vein
- vesical plexus

Lymph Drainage

- internal/communal/external iliac nodes
- lumbar nodes
- renal lymph nodes

Innervation

- sympathetic nervous system from T10 to L1 via the lesser and lowest splanchnic nerves and the lumbar splanchnic nerves 1 and 2 to the celiac plexus, aorticorenal ganglion, renal plexus, and posterior renal ganglion
- vagus nerve (via the celiac plexus)
- sacral parasympathetic system (S2–S4) via the superior hypogastric plexus to the renal plexus

Movement Physiology according to Barral

Mobility

The urinary bladder moves together with the sacrum and uterus: during inhalation posteriorly and superiorly and during exhalation anteriorly and inferiorly.

Another movement results when the bladder is filled with urine and then voided.

Motility

During the expiratory phase, we see a movement posterosuperiorly, and during the inspiratory phase in the opposite direction.

Physiology

Mechanism of Bladder Filling and Voiding

Urine reaches the bladder in portions. The peristaltic contraction of the ureter opens and closes the opening of the ureter.

The ureter penetrates the urinary bladder diagonally. As a result, the internal pressure of the bladder keeps the entrance of the ureter closed except for during peristaltic waves. This mechanism prevents a reflux of urine.

Micturition

The pelvic floor becomes limp, and the bladder consequently shifts lower, its neck assuming a funnel shape.

Urine enters the urethra up to the inner sphincter, the detrusor muscle of the bladder contracts (innervated parasympathetically), and the funnel shape is reinforced. The sphincter opens.

The urethra muscles and the external sphincter become limp.

To conclude micturition, the pelvic floor as well as the internal and external sphincter contract, and the neck of the bladder loses its funnel shape.

Pathologies

Symptoms that Require Medical Clarification

- Hematuria
- Dysfunctions/changes in micturition

Cystitis

Definition. Infection of the upper urinary tract due to pathogenic organisms.

Causes. Highly virulent organisms coinciding with a weakened state of defense.

Precipitating factors include:
- stricture of the urinary tract, e.g., prostatic hyperplasia
- vesicoureteral reflux
- neurogenic disturbance of bladder voiding
- calculi
- diabetes mellitus
- immunosuppressive therapy

Clinical
- dysuria
- pollakiuria
- subfebrile temperatures

Osteopathic Practice

Cardinal Symptoms

- Hematuria
- Dysfunctions/changes in micturition

Typical Dysfunctions

Ptosis

Possible causes include:
- loss of elasticity in the pelvic floor due to pregnancy, age, or depression
- pressure from the organs located superiorly due to abdominal ptosis

Adhesions

Possible causes include surgical operations, e.g., cesarean section.

Spasms

Possible cause is recurrent cystitis.

Associated Structural Dysfunctions

- sacrum
- sacrococcygeal joint
- symphysis
- T7 and T11
- L1 or L2
- proximal and distal tibiofibular joint (chain from obturator internus via the sacrospinal and sacrotuberal ligaments to biceps femoris)

Atypical Symptoms

A list of symptoms follows that can be explained by means of osteopathic chains or result from the patient's history (for an explanation of osteopathic chains, see "Atypical Symptoms" in Chapter 5, page 39):
- recurrent pain and blockages at the lumbosacral transition
- feeling of "breaking through" in the lower lumbar spinal column (LSC) and in the area of the iliosacral joint
- bladder spasms precipitated by spinal column extension and maximum arm lifting

Indications for Osteopathic Treatment

- ptosis with incontinence after coughing, sneezing, laughing, or urinary dribbling
- recurrent cystitis after ruling out anatomic strictures
- disturbed bladder voiding due to scars or prostatic hyperplasia
- vesicoureteral reflux
- bladder stones (require proceeding with caution and gentleness—risk of injury!)

Contraindications for Osteopathic Treatment

- pregnancy
- catheter
- intrauterine device (IUD)
- hematuria
- acute cystitis

Notes for Clinical Application

When seen as a functional cycle, the lesser pelvis brings the four pillars of osteopathy closer together than any other region of the body. Here, we find parietal, visceral, craniosacral, and fascial structures that are functionally interconnected in a unique way.

Parietal or structural osteopathy is concerned with the locomotor system. In functional terms, the pelvis is treated as the LPH (lumbus–pelvis–hip) region in manual therapy and osteopathy. This fact already shows that the pelvis does not exist in isolation but must be viewed in context, by including the hip joint and LSC in our considerations. In turn, this means that these structures of the locomotor system act as a unit, both in terms of physiology and in the case of dysfunctions: if the hip joint is limited in its mobility, this also results in impaired mobility in the iliosacral joint.

The joints are not independent structures; they are surrounded by ligaments and fascia, and they are moved by muscles. These structures are therefore linked to the joints in functional terms: a shortened muscle changes the joint position as well as the range of motion, and a blocked joint leads to hypertonicity in the associated muscles.

Thus, if we consider the locomotor system of the LPH region in isolation, we find numerous ways of explaining dysfunctions in this functional cycle.

In the lesser pelvis, several organs such as the urinary bladder, uterus, adnexas, rectum, cecum, sigmoid, prostate, urethra, seminal vesicle, ureter, and a series of smaller reproductive glands are located in close vicinity to each other. Most of these are in direct contact with more than two other organs of the lesser pelvis. In addition, they are connected to each other by ligaments and fascia: deep inside the lesser pelvis, immediately above the muscular floor of the pelvis, an attachment line runs in an anteroposterior direction, connecting the urinary bladder, uterus/prostate, and rectum to each other. This is the pubovesico-uterorectosacral lamina or Delbet lamina. It consists of the following ligaments: pubovesical, vesicouterine, rectouterine, sacrouterine, and rectosacral. This lamina interconnects the organs of the lesser pelvis in functional terms; consequently, as in the locomotor system, a dysfunction in one organ leads to a disturbance of another organ in this anteroposterior progression. Hence we must never isolate these organs from each other!

It is also important to note that the Delbet lamina is inserted anteriorly into the pubis and posteriorly into the sacrum. In this way, the osseous pelvic ring is included in this chain in functional terms, and any movement impairment in an organ also affects the pubis and sacrum. One example: a cesarean section has resulted in adhesions in the lesser pelvis with impaired mobility in the uterus. At the same time, recurrent blockages occur in the sacrum because the sacrum is no longer able to move freely and the uterus is restricted in its movements. If we now treat only the iliosacral joint and forget about visceral treatment, we will not change the condition as a whole.

In addition, however, the Delbet lamina must be considered in an even larger context: it is the caudal endpoint of the central tendon, i.e., the fascial cord that runs all the way through the body from the base of the skull to the floor of the pelvis. It acts as a functional unit: the entire central tendon accommodates dysfunctions by means of fascial contractions in such a way that the disturbed area of the body is protected to the greatest extent possible. If the lamina is included in this fascial contraction of the central tendon, tensions and movement disorders can arise in its entire anteroposterior chain. Recurrent bladder infections, symphysis pain, and pain in the lumbosacral transition are some of the possible results.

The organs of the lesser pelvis have even more interesting connections to the parietal pelvic ring. Thus, the broad ligament of the uterus is inserted into the ilium via the iliac fascia and the iliacus. This transverse line of fixation in the lesser pelvis is connected via the uterus to the Delbet lamina and functions in a similar manner: if the organ is disturbed, a malposition of the ilium can result. How many cases of pelvic obliquity could in this context receive a different explanation than a purely orthopedic one?

The connections from the lesser pelvis extend even further cranially: the coccyx is a highly mobile bone and adapts with great flexibility to tensions and tissue pulls that affect it. Thus we frequently find malpositions of the coccyx in the frontal plane, but also in the sagittal plane with a sharp bend to anterior.

Although frontal malpositions can be better explained in fascial and muscular terms (i.e., their causes are also found in the lesser pelvis), the main cause of sagittal malposition is traumatic, e.g., a fall. The spinal dura mater inserts itself via its terminal filament into the coccyx. The dura itself is attached in the vertebral canal to the vertebrae S2, C2, and C3, as well as to the foramen magnum. Chronic malpositions of the coccyx are transmitted to the unstretchable dura as tissue tensions up into the upper cervical spinal column (CSC) and the skull. Malpositions of the head joints or headaches can hence also be explained by the functional cycle "lesser pelvis."

The obturator internus likewise has significant topographic relationships to two organs of the lesser pelvis, namely the urinary bladder and the ovary. With its ventrolateral wall, the bladder directly abuts the obturator foramen and thereby the obturator internus. If this organ is affected by adhesions, spasms, or ptosis, the effects can be seen in this muscle. Anatomically, we even find frequent fascial–ligamentary connections between the bladder and obturator internus. As a result of the organic dysfunction and its close topographic relationship to the bladder, the muscle becomes hypertonic and can be palpated at the obturator foramen. It is also common that this tension is felt on only one side—a good diagnostic sign for the disturbed side of the bladder or of the entire lesser pelvis.

The ovary lies in the ovarian fossa, which is bordered laterally by the obturator internus. This organ can also irritate the muscle, when, for example, a cyst, an inflammation, or adhesions after surgery have impaired the organ. Moreover, the obturator nerve lies caudal in the depression of the ovary. If this nerve is irritated by a pathologic ovary, this can manifest as knee pain. A sensitive time for this type of knee pain is puberty in young women. The incipient hormonal cycle triggers movement in the reproductive organs of the lesser pelvis. The ovaries and fallopian tubes perform the necessary rotations and longitudinal shifts to accept the egg via the tubes after ovulation. These monthly recurrent movements did not take place for the first 10–12 years of life; now they have to become attuned to each other, the necessary structures must stretch and free themselves from their previous positions. As a result, tensions arise on the structures that border directly on the ovary, affecting the obturator nerve in particular by irritating it; this manifests as knee pain. In treatment, we should hence concentrate on the lesser pelvis and not try to treat the knee.

Another topographic relationship of great interest can develop between the ovary and piriformis, in cases when the ovary—as in women who have had several pregnancies—has slid far posteriorly and caudally. In such cases, irritation can result, with hypertonicity in the muscle similar to that in the obturator internus—the well-known piriformis syndrome.

Let us turn to the circulation of the organ, because here we also find several special characteristics compared with other areas of the body. The internal iliac artery supplies the pelvic organs arterially. In this area, it is not the case that a single branch of this artery exclusively supplies just one organ; the branches of the artery cover the organs of the lesser pelvis similarly to a root system, and one organ receives blood from several branches. This means that arterial circulation again consolidates the organs into one functional unit. It is also for this reason that the organs must not be separated from each other: if you want to treat them via the circulatory system, you cannot treat just one organ in isolation; this treatment always affects all the other organs in the lesser pelvis. The same holds true for the venous supply of these organs as well: different plexus and central veins lead the blood into the internal iliac vein—where a functional unit is also established.

Lastly, we must mention innervation. There are three vegetative plexus in the lesser pelvis: the superior hypogastric plexus at the height of L5–S1, i.e., at the entrance into the lesser pelvis; the sacral plexus in front of the sacrum; and the inferior hypogastric plexus, which covers the pelvic organs similarly to a spider's web. In contrast to the intra- and retroperitoneal organs, which receive their innervation via the arteries, here a web of nerve fibers around the organs forms independent nerves separate from the arteries, which again interconnect the organs on a functional level. Segmentally, the organs are supplied sympathetically from T10 to L2 and parasympathetically from S2 to S4. Through segmental reflexes at the spinal cord level, irritation of the organs in the lesser pelvis can be transformed as afferent sensory information in the spinal cord into efferent motoric impulses. As a result, hypertonicity develops in the corresponding segmental muscles. For the organs of the lesser pelvis, these are the following muscles:

- erector spinae
- rectus abdominis
- external oblique
- internal oblique
- transversus abdominis
- pyramidalis
- quadratus lumborum
- iliopsoas
- obturator internus
- pelvic floor muscles
- piriformis
- adductor group of the thigh

Complaints that can result from a dysfunction of these muscles manifest among other symptoms as:

- pseudoischialgia
- medial idiopathic knee pain
- blockages of the iliosacral joint
- capsular pattern of the hip joint
- coccydynia
- acute lumbalgia
- acute lumboischialgia
- recurrent pulling of the adductors
- piriformis syndrome

A careful analysis of the visceral aspect of the lesser pelvis can hence make much parietal therapy unnecessary.

Osteopathic Tests and Treatment

Test and Treatment of Bladder Mobility Cranially in the Supine Position according to Barral

Starting Position
The patient is in the supine position, legs bent. The practitioner stands next to the patient.

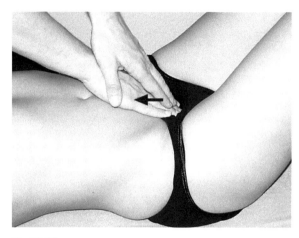

Fig. 15.10

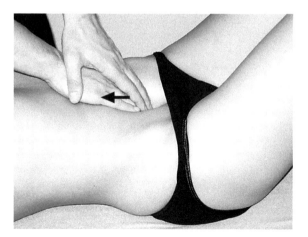

Fig. 15.11

Testing Procedure for the Median Umbilical Ligament
Place the fingers of both hands slightly superior and on both sides lateral to the symphysis onto the abdominal wall. Initially apply pressure posteriorly, then pull superiorly, thereby lifting the urinary bladder cranially.

Next, position the fingers slightly further cranially on both sides of the median line on the abdominal wall and repeat the test. Proceed likewise all the way to the navel.

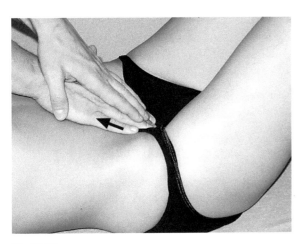

Fig. 15.12

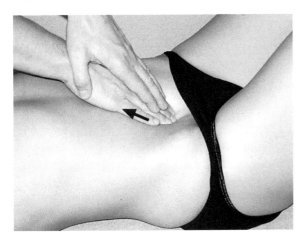

Fig. 15.13

Both tests can also be performed with the patient in a seated position.

Mobilization Cranially in the Seated Position according to Barral

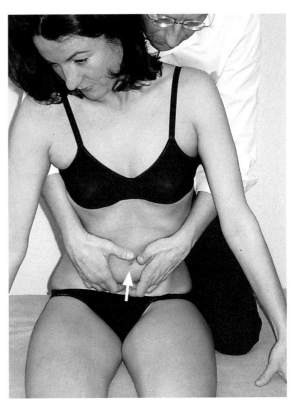

Fig. 15.14

Testing Procedure for Medial Umbilical Ligaments
Position the fingers slightly further laterally to the symphysis on the abdominal wall. Initially, apply pressure posteriorly and then pull superomedially.

Subsequently move along the course of the ligament slightly craniomedially and test at a different place.

In this way, identify painful areas of the ligaments and atypical tensions.

Treatment
Place both hands on the abdominal wall at the median line between symphysis and navel and apply pressure posteriorly and superiorly. Stretching the median umbilical ligament exerts a mobilizing pull on the bladder and mobilizes the ligament as well.

Diverse starting points between symphysis and navel are possible.

If you place your fingers to the right and left of the median line, you can reach the medial umbilical ligaments by pressure posteriorly. The mobilizing pull is performed superomedially, in accordance with the course of the ligaments.

Starting Position
The patient sits in a kyphotic position. The practitioner stands behind the patient.

Procedure
With both hands, make contact with the abdominal wall on the median line and apply pressure posteriorly, to fixate the median umbilical ligament. While maintaining this fixation point, straighten out the patient, thereby causing a pull on the urinary bladder cranially. Repeat this rhythmically.

The fixed points can be positioned at various locations on the line symphysis–navel.

This technique also has an effect on the uterus and prostate.

Mobilization of the Pubovesical Ligament according to Barral

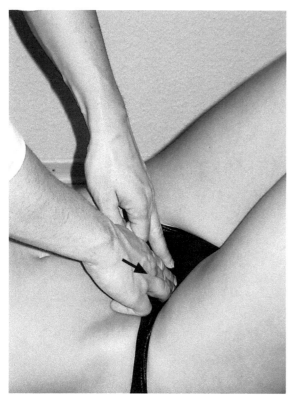

Fig. 15.15

Starting Position
The patient is in the supine position, legs bent. The practitioner stands next to the patient at shoulder level.

Procedure
Position the fingers of both hands to the right and left of the median line directly above the pubic bone next to the symphysis, pushing the skin lightly—the fingers pointing caudally.

Apply light pressure posteriorly and inferiorly, thereby arriving between the urinary bladder and the pubic bone (retropubic space).

It is important to apply pressure with great care because this procedure can be very painful if forced. Hold this gentle pressure until you sense a release in the structures—the sensitivity decreases at the same time.

In this manner, move your fingers step by step medially.

Combined Technique for the Median Umbilical Ligament, Medial Umbilical Ligament, and Pubovesical Ligament in the Supine Position according to Barral

Starting Position
The patient is in the supine position, legs bent. The practitioner stands next to the patient at the height of the pelvis.

Procedure
Place your cranial hand on the abdominal wall:
1. For the median umbilical ligament, on a line symphysis–navel, exert pressure posteriorly.

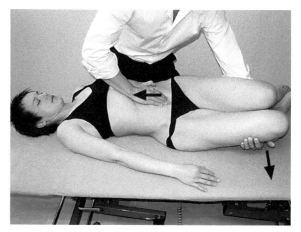

Fig. 15.16

2. For the medial umbilical ligaments, slightly lateral of the median line on the path of the ligament from lateral–caudal to medial–cranial, exert pressure posteriorly.

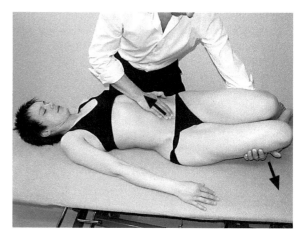

Fig. 15.17

3. For the pubovesical ligament, above the pubic bone and lateral to the symphysis the pressure is in a caudal–posterior direction.

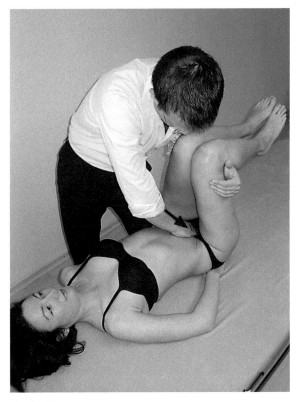

Fig. 15.18

Treatment
With the caudal hand, guide the legs into ipsi- or contralateral rotation (move the knee toward the table). The cranial hand holds or increases the pull caused by this movement.

The more the hips are flexed, the deeper the mobilization of the pubovesical ligament can be performed.

Combined Technique for Stretching the Ureter in the Seated Position according to Barral

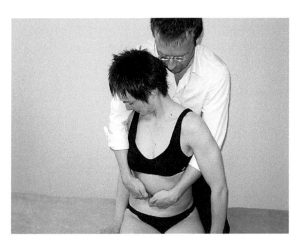

Fig. 15.19

Starting Position
The patient sits in a kyphotic position. The practitioner stands behind the patient.

Procedure
Make contact with the lower pole of the kidney (see above) and fixate the kidney. Lead the patient into extension and ipsilateral rotation and stretch the ureter. Repeat this rhythmically.

Ureter Mobilization via the Peritoneum

By partially fixating the ureter on the posterior peritoneum, peritoneal techniques have a good effect on the ureter. In particular the general relief technique is recommended (see above).

Obturator Foramen Technique

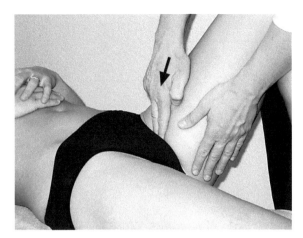

Fig. 15.20

Starting Position
The patient is in the supine position, legs bent. The practitioner stands on the side to be examined.

Procedure
Let the patient's ipsilateral leg lean against your abdomen and hold it fixated with your caudal hand. Guide your cranial hand on the medial side of the thigh along the long adductor muscle group cranially up to the pectineus.

There, position the thumb and exert pressure with the thumb medially and posteriorly, until you reach the obturator externus at the obturator foramen. There, treat by inhibition or vibration.

Variation
For a second path of access to the obturator foramen, place your thumb posterior to the adductor muscle group on the pubic bone and palpate forward craniolaterally

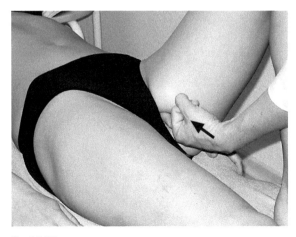

Fig. 15.21

until you reach the obturator externus anterior to the obturator foramen.

This technique has a good circulatory effect on the pelvic organs.

Test and Treatment of Motility

Of the Urinary Bladder according to Barral

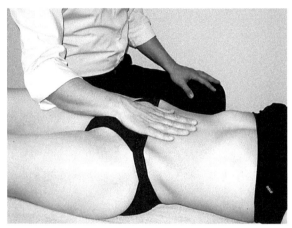

Fig. 15.22

Starting Position
The patient is in the supine position. The practitioner sits next to the patient at the level of the thigh.

Procedure
Place one hand with the thenar right above the symphysis on the median line, with the fingers pointing cranially.

Testing Sequence
Detect the motility movement: during the expiratory phase, you can notice a movement posterosuperiorly to the navel; during the inspiratory phase the movement is in the opposite direction.

Evaluate the amplitude and direction of the inspiratory and expiratory movements as well as the rhythm of the movement as a whole. If a disturbance is present in one or both aspects of the motility movement, treat the patient.

Treatment
Motility is treated indirectly by following the unimpaired movement, remaining at the end-point of this movement for several cycles, and then following the impaired movement to the new end-point.

You can also try to increase the range of the free movement (induction), afterward checking whether the limited movement direction has improved.

Repeat this movement again and again until the motility has returned to normal in terms of rhythm, direction, and amplitude.

Of Bladder and Sacrum Simultaneously according to Barral

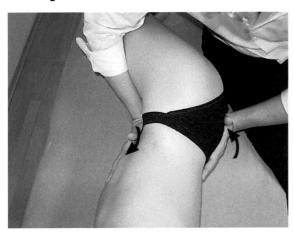

Fig. 15.23

Starting Position

The patient is in the lateral position, legs bent. The practitioner stands next to the patient at the height of the knee.

Procedure

Place one hand with the thenar right above the symphysis on the median line, with the fingers pointing cranially. The palm of the caudal hand makes contact with the sacrum, fingers pointing cranially.

Testing Sequence

Detect the motility movement: the cranial hand moves during the expiratory phase posterosuperiorly, the caudal hand at the same time anteroinferiorly—and back in the inspiratory phase. Evaluate the amplitude and direction of the inspiratory and expiratory movements as well as the rhythm of the movement as a whole. If a disturbance is present in one or both aspects of the motility movement, treat the patient.

Treatment

Motility is treated indirectly by following the unimpaired movement, remaining at the end-point of this movement for several cycles, and then following the impaired movement to the new end-point.

You can also try to increase the range of the free movement (induction), afterward checking whether the limited movement direction has improved.

Repeat this movement again and again until the motility has returned to normal in terms of rhythm, direction, and amplitude.

Circulatory Techniques according to Kuchera

Arterial Stimulation

- diaphragm techniques
- obturator foramen technique

Venous Stimulation

- liver pump
- diaphragm techniques
- obturator foramen technique

Lymphatic Stimulation

- lymph drainage on thorax and abdomen
- diaphragm techniques

Vegetative Harmonization

Sympathetic nervous system:
- rib raising T12–L2
- inhibiting the paravertebral muscles
- vibrations
- manipulations
- Maitland technique
- stimulating the inferior mesenteric ganglion
- diaphragm techniques

Parasympathetic nervous system:
Stimulation of the vagus nerve for the ureter by:
- craniosacral therapy
- laryngeal techniques
- thoracic techniques (recoil)
- diaphragm techniques.
Stimulation of segments S2–S4 by:
- iliosacral joint techniques
- ischiorectal fossa technique
- pelvic floor technique

Reflex Point Treatment according to Chapman

Location of the Urinary Bladder

Anterior. Around the navel. Slightly lateral of the symphysis, between the two branches of the pubic bone.

Posterior. Upper edge of the tip of the transverse process of L2 (both sides).

Location of the Ureter

Anterior. Inner edge of the superior branch of the pubis, near the upper edge of the symphysis (both sides).

Posterior. Upper edge of the tip of the transverse process of L2 (both sides).

Treatment Principle

Make contact with the reflex point. For this purpose, very gently place a finger on the point and press only lightly. Reflex points are often very sensitive, and it is therefore important to proceed with caution.

The finger remains on the point and treatment is by gentle rotations.

The anterior points are treated first, then the posterior points. Continue with the treatment until you have normalized the sensitivity or consistency of the point.

To conclude, check the anterior points once more. If you fail to notice any change, it is possible that the organ pathology is too great to be influenced quickly via the reflex points, or other dysfunctions are present that must be treated first.

Recommendations for the Patient

The desirable amount of fluids to consume every day is 2–3 L, in addition to food. This is an effective preventive treatment for urinary calculi and bladder infections.

Self-Mobilization of the Urinary Bladder by Fascial Pull on the Urachus

In the supine or head-down position, place the hands on the abdomen above the pubis, press lightly posteriorly, and then pull with both hands cranially in the direction of the navel.

16 The Uterus / Fallopian Tubes / Ovaries

Anatomy

▨ Anatomy of the Uterus

General Facts

- pear shaped
- weight 30–120 g, length 7–9 cm long (nullipara: 6–8 cm)

Function

- Defends against organisms invading the uterine cavity and the abdominal space.
- Ensures the passage of sperm.
- Contains and nourishes the embryo.
- Expels the fetus during childbirth.

Form

- vaginal portion
- cervix
- body
- fundus
- isthmus

Location

Flexion = inclination between longitudinal axis of the cervix and body of the uterus

Normal: anteflexion (axis of the body is almost horizontal when the woman is standing, cervical axis is pointing dorsocaudally)

Version = inclination of the cervical axis to the longitudinal axis

Normal: anteversion (cervical axis is tipped forward)

Position = position of the vaginal portion in the pelvic space

Normal: vagina at the height of the interspinal line in the center of the pelvis or slightly to the left

Factors Affecting the Location

- condition of the uterine support structure
- degree of fullness in the urinary bladder and rectum
- processes of shrinking and displacement in the lesser pelvis

Projection onto the Wall of the Torso

- lower third of the uterus: immediately above the symphysis
- supravaginal part of the cervix: sacrococcygeal joint

Topographic Relationships

- peritoneum
- urinary bladder
- rectum
- vagina
- small intestinal loops
- sigmoid colon
- fallopian tube
- ovary
- ureter
- uterine artery and vein

Attachments / Suspensions

- pelvic floor (levator ani)
- suspensory ligament of the ovary–proper ligament of the ovary–round ligament of the uterus
- broad ligaments/plica lata
- sacrouterine and rectouterine ligaments
- vesicouterine ligament

Circulation

Arterial

Uterine artery (from the internal iliac artery) anastomosed with the ovarian artery (from the aorta).

Venous

Uterine vein and diverse plexus that run into the internal iliac vein.

Lymph Drainage

- lumbar lymph nodes
- superficial inguinal lymph nodes
- external iliac lymph nodes
- obturator lymph nodes

Innervation

- sympathetic nervous system from T10 to L2 via the splanchnic nerves to the celiac/superior and inferior mesenteric ganglions and renal plexus
- With vessels (ovarian artery) or as independent nerve fibers, the nerves run to the hypogastric and utero-vaginal plexus.
- Postganglionic supply from the four sacral ganglions and the ganglion impar is under discussion.

Sacral parasympathetic nervous system (S2–S4) to the inferior hypogastric plexus and uterovaginal plexus

▦ Anatomy of the Ovaries

General Facts

- Size: 4 cm long, 2 cm wide, 1 cm thick.
- Weight: 6–8 g.

Function

The ovaries are the female sex glands. In addition, they produce estrogens, progestogens, and steroids.

Location

In the standing female, the ovaries lie on top of the broad ligament (posterior) and between the suspensory ligament of the ovary and the proper ligament of the ovary in an infolding of peritoneum.

The longitudinal axis runs virtually craniocaudal.

The ovary sits higher in nulliparas than in multiparas. It lies in a depression (ovarian fossa) with borders formed by the following structures:

- obturator internus (lateral)
- external iliac vein (anterior)
- umbilical artery, obturator artery, obturator nerve (caudal)
- ureter, internal iliac vessels (cranioposterior)

Topographic Relationships

- ovarian fossa
- peritoneum
- psoas fascia (via the insertion of the suspensory ligament of the ovary)
- ileum
- ovarian vessels
- uterine artery
- cecum (right ovary)
- appendix (right ovary)
- piriformis (in multiparas)
- obturator nerve

Projection onto the Wall of the Torso

The ovaries project onto the abdominal wall in a line on the anterosuperior iliac spine (ASIS)—upper edge of the symphysis, slightly medial to the edge of the psoas.

Attachments/Suspensions

- Suspensory ligament of the ovary (from ovary to ileum and psoas fascia): this ligament leads the ovarian vessels and nerves to the ovary.
- Proper ligament of the ovary (from ovary to angle of the tube): it contains a branch of the uterine artery.
- Peritoneal cover with mesovarium: it also covers the two upper ligaments.

Circulation

Arterial

- uterine artery (from the internal iliac artery)
- ovarian artery (aorta)

Venous

- ovarian vein: on the right drains into the inferior vena cava; on the left drains into the left renal vein and then
- inferior vena cava
- uterine vein and diverse plexus that run into the internal iliac vein

Lymph Drainage

Lumbar lymph nodes.

Innervation

- sympathetically, the ovaries are supplied by the same segments as the uterus.
- vagus nerve

Movement Physiology according to Barral

Mobility

The uterus is highly mobile, its position dependent on the menstrual cycle, the state of fullness in the urinary bladder and rectum, and the position of the small intestinal loops.

Filled Urinary Bladder

The uterus is pressed posteriorly.

Filled Rectum

The uterus is pressed anteriorly.

Filled Rectum and Urinary Bladder

The uterus is pressed superiorly.

Pregnancy

The uterus is pressed inferiorly.

Lateral displacement occurs as the result of scarring.

The fallopian tubes are also very mobile: the fimbriae perform rhythmic movements in three planes at the start of ovulation.

To transport the oocyte, we see both segmental and peristaltic contractions of the entire fallopian tube as well as movements of the fimbriae and cilia in the tube.

The position of the ovary depends on the movements of the uterus.

Motility

Uterus

Similar to the urinary bladder: during the expiratory phase, we see a movement posterosuperiorly; during the inspiratory phase the movement is in the opposite direction.

Ovary

Left ovary: rotation in a clockwise direction and slightly superior.

Right ovary: rotation in a counterclockwise direction and slightly superior.

Physiology

The reproductive hormones are subject to a hormonal regulatory circuit with the hypothalamus, hypophysis, and ovaries serving as hormonal glands.

Hypothalamus

The hypothalamus produces luteinizing hormone (LH)-releasing hormone (LHRH), which stimulates the adenohypophysis to produce and release gonadotropic hormones.

Hypophysis

Follicle-Stimulating Hormone

The follicle-stimulating hormone (FSH) has the following effects in the ovary:
- maturation of the follicles
- formation of estradiol receptors
- production of estradiol from testosterone (in the testicles, it stimulates spermatogenesis)

Luteinizing Hormone

The luteinizing hormone (LH) has the following effects in the ovary:
- production of estrogen and progesterone
- changes in the follicular wall that lead to ovulation (in the testicles, it stimulates testosterone synthesis)

Human chorionic gonadotropin (hCG) in the placenta roughly corresponds to LH.

Hormones of the Ovaries

Estrogens

Most estrogens are formed in the ovary. The starting molecule is cholesterol, which through several intermediary steps is transformed into testosterone. This is then turned into estradiol in yet another conversion. Estrogens are also produced in other tissues from androgens (see below), and they are also formed in the testicles.

The phase of estrogen production coincides with the phase of follicular maturation.

The effect is as follows:
- stimulates growth of the female reproductive organs
- regeneration and growth of the endometrium
- secretion of thin, spinnable, clear, alkaline mucus (facilitates the inflow of sperm)
- promotes the movement of the fallopian tubes and their production of secretions
- epithelial growth in the vagina; also partially responsible for a normal vaginal environment

- stimulates the growth of the mammary glands
- formation of subcutaneous fat deposits (female body shape)
- promotes formation of secondary sexual characteristics (growth of pubic hair, pigmentation of the nipples and vulva)
- lifts the mood

Progesterone

This is formed only in the ovaries and placenta from cholesterol. Progesterone production occurs during the luteal phase.

The effect is as follows:
- transforms the endometrium which is proliferating under the influence of estrogen
- production of thick cervical mucus that is impermeable to sperm
- epithelial cells in the vagina are discharged repeatedly
- lowers tonicity in the uterine muscles and reduces uterine contractions—immobilizes the uterus during pregnancy
- under the influence of progesterone, we see a general drop in tonicity of the smooth muscles
- stimulates the growth of the mammary glands
- progesterone causes a rise in body temperature of 0.4–0.6 °C

In conclusion, we can say that estrogens prepare the body for conception and progesterone prepares it for pregnancy.

Ovarian Cycle

Follicular Maturation

In a negative feedback response, the drop of progesterone in the corpus luteum after menstruation causes an increased release of FSH in the hypophysis.

As a result, several follicles mature.

Recruitment Phase

LH and FSH stimulate the production of estrogens in the follicles. The high estrogen level causes a drop in FSH release, which leads to the destruction of most follicles before they have matured.

Selection Phase

The follicle with the greatest maturity reaches ovulation because it does not depend on external FSH due to its internal amount of FSH and estrogens, and it therefore continues to grow.

Ovulation

A peak in LH and the start of progesterone production induce the release of the oocyte from the ruptured follicle.

Luteal Phase

Under the influence of FSH and LH, the corpus luteum produces estrogens and progesterone. If no fertilization takes place, the corpus luteum begins to disintegrate after 10–12 days.

If fertilization has taken place, however, the corpus luteum continues to have a function. The fertilized egg produces hCG and thereby stimulates continued hormone production in the corpus luteum.

Cycle of the Uterine Mucosa

Proliferation Phase

After menstruation, estrogens cause the growth of a new mucous membrane. This takes approximately 10 days.

Secretory Phase

Progesterone stimulates glandular growth in the new mucosa with the production of large amounts of secretions.

Menstruation

If fertilization does not occur, the progesterone level drops due to the deterioration of the corpus luteum. This missing hormonal stimulus changes the metabolism and circulation in the uterine mucosa, which at last leads to rupture-induced bleeding and fibrinolysis. As a result of the fibrinolysis, menstrual blood does not coagulate. The average loss of blood is 30–80 mL.

Regeneration

Due to the effect of estrogen, the surface of the wound is closed again.

Menopause

Most women experience the great hormonal changes of this period of life between the ages of 45 and 55. There are large organic changes, manifesting in a multitude of symptoms.

In the ovaries, change already occurs in the fourth decade of a woman's life: scleroses of vessels, decrease in the number of follicles, and lowered response to hormones from the hypophysis. As a result, cycles can occur without ovulation, which explains why it becomes more difficult from the mid-40s on to become pregnant.

When all the follicles have deteriorated, the ovary stops producing estrogen.

The following are the possible effects of estrogen deficiency:
- vegetative symptoms such as heat flashes, dizziness, palpitations, sweating, paraesthesia
- disturbances in normal menstrual bleeding before the onset of the menopause
- atrophic changes in the mucous membranes of the genitalia: loss of elasticity, dry thin skin, greater vulnerability, shrinkage
- changes in the skin: thin, dry, wrinkled
- arteriosclerosis (female hormones have a preventive effect on vascular diseases)
- osteoporosis
- Psychological changes such as depression, irritability, sleeping disorders, or nervousness should be not only attributed to the hormone deficiency, but also regarded as the result of the experienced bodily changes and the thought processes involved in coming to terms with these.
- incontinence
- organ ptoses (bladder, uterus)

Pathologies

Symptoms that Require Medical Clarification

- Vaginal bleeding independent of the menstrual cycle
- Changes in the menstrual period (abnormally strong, prolonged, too frequent, irregular)
- Contact bleeding
- Postmenopausal bleeding
- Pre- or postmenstrual spotting
- Discharge (previously unknown, dark, foul smelling)
- Feeling of having a foreign body in the lower abdomen
- Previously unknown bladder complaints, problems or pain with defecation

Myoma

Definition. Benign tumor of the uterine muscles; deterioration is possible.

Causes. Estrogens seem to cause the excessive growth in the muscles.

Symptoms. Symptoms depend on localization, size, direction of growth, and number of myomas. Accordingly, the following symptoms are possible:
- changes in menstruation (prolonged, increased, intermenstrual bleeding, different patterns of pain)

- pattern of an acute abdomen
- frequent urinary urgency
- impaired intestinal voiding
- fertility disorders

Endometriosis

Definition. Presence of hormonally regulated tissue similar to uterine mucosa outside the uterine cavity.

Causes. Retrograde menstruation through the fallopian tubes and adhesion of endometrial tissue outside the uterus.

Symptoms. Depending on the localization of the tissue, we see different symptoms:
- cyclical pain (most commonly 1–3 days before menstruation and receding at the peak of the menstrual period)
- increased, prolonged menstrual periods
- sterility
- tubal pregnancy
- ovarian cysts
- adhesions to the surroundings
- lumbalgia

Salpingitis/Oophoritis

Definition. Inflammation of the fallopian tubes/ovaries.

Causes. Infection from pathogenic organisms due to:
- spreading upward via the vagina and uterus
- transmission from the surroundings (e.g., appendix)
- hematogenous transmission (e.g., tuberculosis, typhoid, viral)

Symptoms
- lower abdominal pain
- fever
- intermenstrual bleeding
- urinary dysfunctions
- bilateral inflammation, but symptoms are often dominant on one side

Osteopathic Practice

Cardinal Symptoms

> - Pain independent of the cycle and menstruation
> - Vaginal bleeding or discharge

Typical Dysfunctions

Adhesions/Fixations

Possible causes include:
- surgery
- infections
- tubal pregnancy
- miscarriage

Ptosis

Possible causes include:
- loss of elasticity due to pregnancy
- obstetric procedures (vacuum extractor, large episiotomy)
- age-related loss of elasticity

Spasms

Possible causes include:
- infections
- psychosomatic
- when the openings of the tubes are occluded, spasms can be the cause of fertility or ovulatory disorders

Circulatory Stasis in the Lesser Pelvis

Possible causes include:
- adhesions/fixations
- ptosis of the small intestine

Associated Structural Dysfunctions

- lumbosacral transition
- reflectory knee pain (topographic closeness to the obturator nerve)
- upper CSC
- T12–L1
- occiput–temporal on the right
- proximal and distal tibiofibular joints
- navicular bone

Atypical Symptoms

A list of symptoms follows that can be explained by means of osteopathic chains or result from the patient's history (for an explanation of osteopathic chains, see "Atypical Symptoms" in Chapter 5, page 39):
- discomfort in the lower abdomen
- lumbalgia
- dysmenorrhea
- disturbed ovulation
- hemorrhoids
- varicose veins
- recurrent cystitis

Indications for Osteopathic Treatment

- see "Atypical Symptoms"
- surgery on the urogenital system
- cesarean section
- episiotomy
- intestinal surgery, e.g., appendectomy
- menopausal symptoms

Contraindications for Osteopathic Treatment

- pregnancy
- IUD
- infections
- obvious painful palpatory findings that cannot be relieved by osteopathic treatment and sometimes even persist unabated for several days after the treatment

Notes for Clinical Application

See "Lesser Pelvis," pages 156–158.

Osteopathic Tests and Treatment

Test and Treatment of the Fundus of the Uterus according to Barral

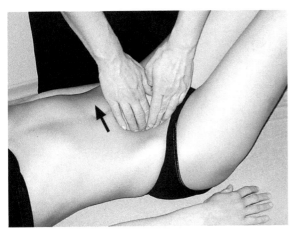

Fig. 16.1

Variation
Unilateral application of this technique is also possible, and you can achieve excellent results in the lateral position.

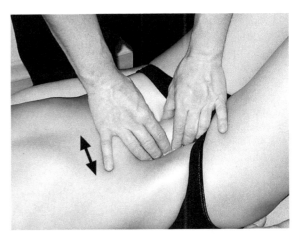

Fig. 16.2

Starting Position
The patient is in the supine position, legs bent, held passively by the practitioner. The practitioner stands next to the patient.

Procedure
Place your hand on the abdominal wall slightly above the symphysis contralateral to the area where rectus abdominis is attached.

With cautious pressure posteriorly, reach the area lateral to the fundus of the uterus.

Testing Sequence
Test the mobility by pulling transversely toward yourself. Take note of sensitivity and atypical tensions.

The more the legs are flexed in the hip, the easier it is to perform this procedure.

Treatment
You can position both hands simultaneously on both sides of the uterus and mobilize the organ in translation. It is important to provide sufficient flexion in the hip to relax the abdominal wall.

Test and Treatment of the Ovaries and Broad Ligament of the Uterus according to Barral

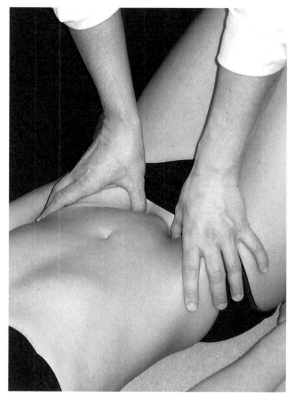

Fig. 16.3

Starting Position

The patient is in the supine position, legs bent. The practitioner stands next to the patient.

Procedure

Visualize the projection of the ovary on the abdominal wall (see above) and place your hand on the abdomen on a line ASIS–symphysis (upper edge), slightly medial to the edge of the psoas.

Slide your hand slowly into the depth posteriorly until you reach the test region. Test the elasticity by comparing sides. Take note of sensitivity and atypical tensions.

As this area tends to be very sensitive, always proceed with caution!

Treatment

You can now cause relaxation of this ligament by means of inhibitions, vibrations, or small rebounds.

Variation

This technique can also be applied unilaterally in the lateral position.

Mobilization of the Uterus via the Median and Medial Umbilical Ligaments in the Supine Position according to Barral

These techniques are described in Chapter 15, pages 158–159. After improving the mobility of the urinary bladder, these also allow you to evaluate and treat the mobility between the urinary bladder and the uterus.

> **Note**
> In general, we can say that any test or treatment of one of these two organs always affects the other one.

Combined Mobilization of the Uterus with Leg Lever in the Supine Position according to Barral

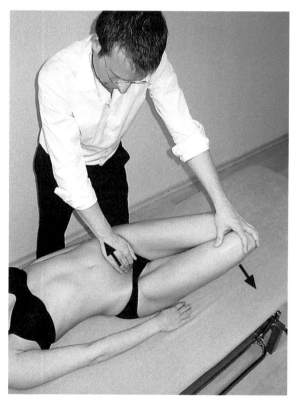

Fig. 16.4

Starting Position

The patient is in the supine position, legs bent. The practitioner stands next to the patient at the level of the pelvis.

Procedure

Position your cranial hand in such a way that you can reach the fundus of the uterus or the broad ligament of the uterus contralaterally. With your caudal hand, hold the patient's legs.

Treatment

With the medial hand, mobilize the uterus medially and fix it there, while guiding the patient's legs away from you with your caudal hand, until the stretch reaches the uterus (place the knee on the table).

In case of a vesicouterine ptosis, the cranial hand can additionally exert a mobilizing pull superiorly.

Obturator Foramen Technique

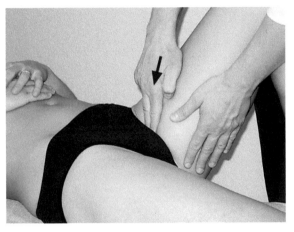

Fig. 16.5

Starting Position

The patient is in the supine position, legs bent. The practitioner stands on the side to be examined.

Procedure

Let the patient's ipsilateral leg lean against your abdomen and hold it there with your caudal hand. Guide your cranial hand on the medial side of the thigh along the long adductor muscle group cranially up to the pectineus.

There, position the thumb and exert pressure with the thumb medially and posteriorly, until you reach the obturator externus at the obturator foramen. Treat here by inhibition or vibrations.

Variation

For a second path of access to the obturator foramen, place your thumb posterior to the adductor muscle group on the pubic bone and palpate forward in a cranial–lateral direction until you reach the obturator externus anterior to the obturator foramen.

This technique has a good circulatory effect on the pelvic organs.

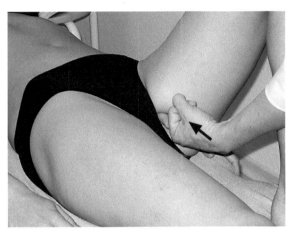

Fig. 16.6

Test and Treatment of Motility according to Barral

Motility of the Uterus

Starting Position

The patient is in the supine position, legs bent. The practitioner stands next to the patient at the level of the thigh.

Procedure

Place one hand with the thenar immediately above the symphysis on the median line, with the fingers pointing cranially.

Testing Sequence

Detect the motility movement: during the expiratory phase, you may notice a movement posterosuperiorly to the navel; during the inspiratory phase this is in the opposite direction. Evaluate the amplitude and direction of the inspiratory and expiratory movements as well as the rhythm of the movement as a whole. If a disturbance is present in one or both aspects of the motility movement, treat the patient.

Treatment

Motility is treated indirectly by following the unimpaired movement, remaining at the end-point of this movement for several cycles, and then following the impaired movement to the new end-point.

You can also try to increase the range of the free movement (induction), afterward checking whether the limited movement direction has improved.

Repeat this movement again and again until the motility has returned to normal in terms of rhythm, direction, and amplitude.

Tubo-Ovarian Motility

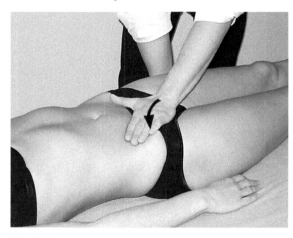

Fig. 16.7

Starting Position

The patient is in the supine position, legs stretched out. The practitioner stands on the contralateral side.

Procedure

Place one hand flat on a line ASIS–symphysis, with the fingers pointing superiorly and slightly laterally.

Test and treatment correspond to the principles described above.

Circulatory Techniques according to Kuchera

Arterial Stimulation

- diaphragm techniques
- obturator foramen technique

Venous Stimulation

- liver pump
- diaphragm techniques
- obturator foramen technique

Lymphatic Stimulation

- lymph drainage on thorax and abdomen
- diaphragm techniques

Vegetative Harmonization—Fallopian Tubes and Ovaries

Sympathetic nervous system:
- rib raising T10–T11
- inhibiting the paravertebral muscles
- vibrations
- manipulations
- Maitland technique
- stimulating the superior mesenteric ganglion
- diaphragm techniques

Parasympathetic nervous system:
Stimulation of the vagus nerve by:
- craniosacral therapy
- laryngeal techniques
- thoracic techniques (recoil)
- diaphragm techniques

Stimulation of segments S2–S4 by:
- iliosacral joint techniques
- ischiorectal fossa technique
- pelvic floor technique

Vegetative Harmonization—Uterus

Sympathetic nervous system:
- rib raising T12–L2
- inhibiting the paravertebral muscles
- vibrations
- manipulations
- Maitland technique
- stimulating the inferior mesenteric ganglion
- diaphragm techniques

Parasympathetic nervous system:
Stimulation of segments S2–S4 by:
- iliosacral joint techniques
- ischiorectal fossa technique
- pelvic floor technique

Reflex Point Treatment according to Chapman

Location for the Uterus

Anterior. On the upper edge of the connection between the superior branch of the pubis and the ischium, lateral to the symphysis (on both sides).

Posterior. Between the posterosuperior iliac spine (PSIS) and the spinous process of L5 (both sides).

Location for the Broad Ligament of the Uterus

Anterior. From the greater trochanter lateral caudally to 5 cm above the knee (on both sides).

Posterior. Between the PSIS and the spinous process of L5 (both sides).

Location for a Myoma

Anterior. Lateral to the symphysis (on both sides).

Posterior. From the tip of the transverse process of L5 approximately 3 cm above the iliac crest, running laterally.

Location for the Ovary

Anterior. Anterior and lateral to the symphysis from the upper to the lower edge (on both sides).

Posterior. Intercostal space between ribs 9–10 and ribs 10–11 on the medial end.

Location for the Ovary/Fallopian Tube

Anterior. Halfway between the acetabulum and ischiadic incisure (on both sides).

Posterior. Between the PSIS and the spinous process of L5 (both sides).

Location for the Prostate Gland

Anterior. From the lateral greater trochanter caudally to 5 cm above the knee (on both sides) and laterally to the symphysis (as for the uterus).

Posterior. Between the PSIS and the spinous process of L5 (both sides).

Treatment Principle

Make contact with the reflex point. For this purpose, very gently place a finger on the point and press only lightly. Reflex points are often very sensitive, so it is important to proceed with caution.

The finger remains on the point and treatment is by gentle rotations.

The anterior points are treated first, then the posterior points. Continue with the treatment until you have normalized the sensitivity or consistency of the point.

To conclude, check the anterior points once more. If you fail to notice any change, it is possible that the organ pathology is too great to be influenced quickly via the reflex points, or other dysfunctions are present that must be treated first.

Recommendations for the Patient

Female Patients with Premenstrual Syndrome

- foods high in tryptophan, e.g., cashew nuts, sunflower seeds, veal, chicken breast
- low-sodium diet
- reduced consumption of alcohol and coffee to a minimum
- diet rich in magnesium (nuts, whole grains, vegetables)
- diet rich in iron (lean meat, raisins, mussels, dark-green vegetables)

Prevention of Osteoporosis and Atherosclerosis

- vitamin D (salmon, tuna fish, Emmental cheese)
- vitamin K (spinach, broccoli, kale, green tea)
- calcium (cheese, sardines, kale, yogurt)
- limited levels of phosphorus (red meat, processed or ready-prepared foods, cola)
- limited intake of coffee, protein, and salt
- limited intake of saturated fats (meat, eggs, whole milk products) and hydrogenated fats (bought baked goods and snacks); favor unsaturated fats (nuts, seeds, and olive oil)
- garlic, ginger, chili peppers, and onions—foods that protect the vessels
- fish, two to three times a week
- antioxidants: citrus fruit, green and yellow vegetables
- Exercise prevents both osteoporosis and atherosclerosis. Suitable forms are endurance sports such as jogging, walking, hiking, cross-country skiing, or inline skating.

17 The Thorax

Anatomy

▨ Anatomy of the Heart

General Facts

The heart is roughly the size of a fist and weighs approximately 300 g.

It is divided by the cardiac septum into a right and a left half, which usually have no connection with each other. In each half, we find an atrium and a ventricle, separated from each other by a flap-shaped valve (atrioventricular or AV valve).

A different type of valve is found in the vessels that lead out of the ventricles—the pocket valves (semilunar valves). Both valves are infoldings of the inner layer of the heart, the endocardium. They function as valves by allowing the inflow of blood in one direction but preventing a backflow in the opposite direction.

Blood Flow in the Body

The oxygen-depleted blood from the body's circulation flows through the superior and inferior vena cavae into the right atrium.

The superior vena cava (SVC) is a central vessel that collects the blood from the upper extremities and the areas of the head and neck. The inferior vena cava (IVC) delivers blood from the abdomen, the lesser pelvis, and the lower extremities.

Through the tricuspid valve, the flap valve of the right heart (three flaps), the blood flows into the right ventricle and from there on through the pulmonary valve into the pulmonary artery. In the capillary net of the lungs, the deoxygenated blood is rearterialized and then flows through the pulmonary veins to the left atrium. After passing through the mitral valve (two flaps), the blood flows into the left ventricle and then on through the aortic valve into the aorta and the rest of the body. The heart functions as a combined pressure-and-suction pump in a closed system.

Layered Structure

The wall of the heart consists of three layers. On the outside is the epicardium, a layer of connective tissue that is followed by the pericardium. The middle layer consists of a meshwork of interconnected striated muscles (syncytium). This special structure guarantees that any impulse in the heart is transmitted from cell to cell.

The muscles of the left ventricle are roughly three times as thick as those of the right ventricle. The reason for this is the difference in pressure that must be built up to expel the blood from the ventricles: the pulmonary circulation is characterized by a pressure of approximately 25 mmHg; the systemic circulation has to overcome a systolic pressure of approximately 120 mmHg. The innermost layer of the heart is the endocardium, which is also formed of connective tissue.

Impulse-Conducting System

The cardiac impulse-conducting system consists of specially built cardiac myocytes that have the ability to autonomously create impulses. The heart's pacemaker is the sinoatrial node, a roughly bean-sized knot at the entrance of the SVC in the right atrium. It generates impulses with a frequency of 70–80/min. After a diffuse transmission through the atria, the AV node receives the impulse. This structure is located at the border between the atrium and ventricle in the right heart. From there, the action potential is conducted to the bundle of His on the right side of the interventricular septum. Then there is a division into two ventricular branches that continue onto the muscles of the right and left ventricles and end in the Purkinje fibers.

Location

The heart is located in the mediastinum inside the pericardium, with the tip pointing toward the front at the bottom left and the base toward the back at the top right. The right half of the heart faces the anterior thoracic wall, the left points posteriorly.

Projection onto the Wall of the Torso

The right border of the heart projects at the sternal attachment of ribs 2–6—approximately 2–3 cm away from the sternum—onto the anterior thoracic wall. The caudal border is formed by the diaphragm.

The left border of the heart runs as follows: cranial for a distance of approximately 2 cm from the sternal attachment of the second rib in a diagonal course to the tip of the heart in the fifth intercostal space approximately 2 cm medial to the medioclavicular line.

Posteriorly, the most caudal point of the heart lies at the level of T10 during exhalation and shifts downward by a distance of one and a half vertebrae during inhalation.

Topographic Relationships

Lateral
- lung, on both sides
- phrenic nerve, on both sides

Anterior
- in the pericardial triangle: sternum
- ribs 2–6
- thymus

Posterior
- spinal column
- esophagus (bordering on the left atrium)
- aorta
- bronchial tubes
- pulmonary artery and vein

Caudal. Diaphragm.

Cranial
- pulmonary artery and vein
- SVC
- aorta

Attachments/Suspensions

Via the pericardium, the heart is firmly attached in the mediastinum. Due to its structure as a serous cavity, the pericardium also ensures frictionless and free moveability during heart activity.

Cranially, the heart is suspended by the entering and exiting vessels.

The pericardium has multiple attachments in all directions:
- Phrenicopericardial ligaments: in the front right, the pericardium is firmly attached to the diaphragm; elsewhere it can be separated bluntly from the diaphragm.
- Sternopericardial ligaments: these run from the pericardium to the manubrium and xiphoid process.
- vertebropericardial ligaments
- cervicopericardial ligaments
- visceropericardial ligaments

There are connections to the esophagus, bronchial tubes, and pulmonary veins.

Laterally, the pericardium is linked via connective tissue to the parietal pleura.

The pericardium and its attachments are incorporated into the fascial system of the "central tendon," which extends from the base of the skull to the lesser pelvis.

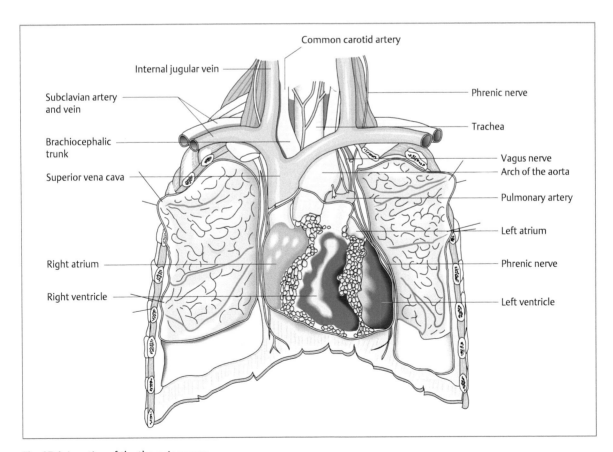

Fig. 17.1 Location of the thoracic organs.

Circulation

A right and a left coronary artery originate at the aortic sinus (dilatation at the origin of the aorta above the aortic valve). During diastole, the pockets of the aortic valve fill up, and blood fills the coronary arteries.

In functional terms, the coronary arteries are end-arteries, i.e., they do not form anastomoses with each other: if a branch of the artery is occluded, the myocardial tissue supplied by this vessel perishes.

Arterial

- left coronary artery:
  - left ventricle
  - anterior wall of the right ventricle
  - ventricular septum
- circumflex branch of the left coronary artery
- both atria
- right coronary artery:
  - right ventricle (majority)
  - ventricular septum

Venous

- Coronary sinus: central vessel for large coronary veins. Leads into the right atrium and drains about two-thirds of all venous blood. Small veins run directly into the cardiac spaces, mostly into the right atrium.

Lymph Drainage

The lymph flows to the anterior mediastinal lymph nodes in front of the tracheal bifurcation and to the lymph nodes in the vicinity of the large vessels by the heart.

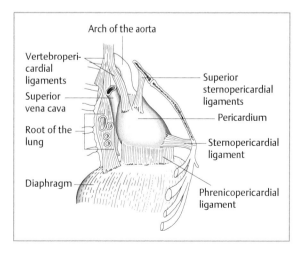

Fig. 17.2 Ligamentous structures of the pericardium.

Innervation

- sympathetic nervous system from T1 to T4
- vagus nerve

Both vegetative sections meet in the cardiac plexus. The plexus surrounds the aorta and the roots of the other large vessels in the vicinity of the heart; from there, vegetative nerves run together with the coronary arteries.

- Phrenic nerve supplies the pericardium sensorily together with the sympathetic and parasympathetic nerves.

Organ Clock

Maximal time: 11 a.m.–1 p.m.
Minimal time: 11 p.m.–1 a.m.

Organ–Tooth Interrelationship

For basic information, see page 34.

> - First incisor in the lower jaw on both sides
> - Second incisor in the upper jaw on both sides

◼ Anatomy of the Lung

General Facts

The two halves of the lung largely fill the lateral chest. The left half of the lung is slightly smaller because the heart claims some of the space in the left chest.

The left half of the lung consists of two lobes that are divided into nine segments. The right half consists of three lobes and ten segments. Each segment is supplied with air by a segmental bronchus. These bronchial tubes combine to form the lobar bronchi, which then form the main bronchus. The two main bronchi together form the trachea.

The actual location of gas exchange is in the alveolae. The human body has approximately 300–400 million alveolae with a total surface area of 100–140 m^2.

The lung is surrounded by the visceral pleura, which runs into the parietal pleura in the suspension area of the lung. The fluid-filled space between the lung and pleura is highly significant for the frictionless mobility and fixation of the lung.

Location

The cavity between the two pleural layers serves partly as extra space into which the lungs can expand during deep inhalations. The borders of the pleura are therefore listed separately from the borders of the lungs.

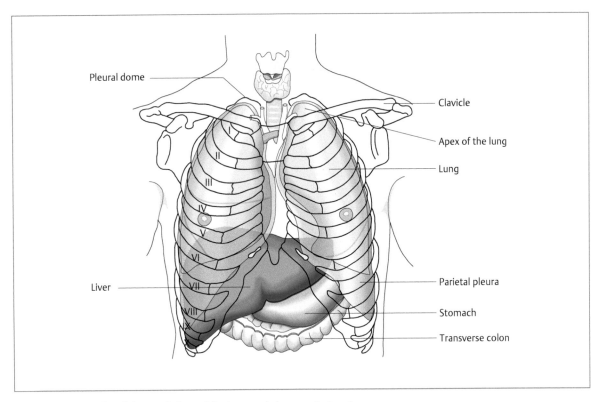

Fig. 17.3 Topography of the two halves of the lung and pleura: anterior view.

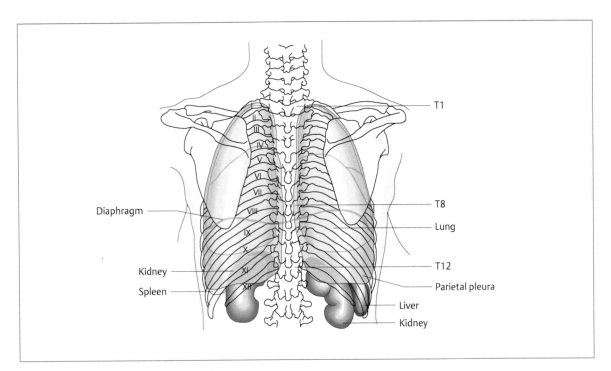

Fig. 17.4 Topography of the two halves of the lung and pleura: posterior view.

Borders of the Pleura

Cranial
Approximately 3 cm above the first rib, tough and thickened.

Anterior and Medial
Behind the sternum, on the left with cardiac impression.

Posterior and Medial
T1–T12, paravertebral.

Caudal
Medioclavicular line:	rib 7
Anterior axillary line:	rib 8
Axillary line:	rib 9
Posterior axillary line:	rib 10
Scapular line:	rib 11
Paravertebral:	rib 12

Borders of the Lung

The cranial and paravertebral borders coincide with those of the pleura. Caudally, the lung sits one or two intercostal spaces above the borders of the pleura during average inhalations.

In deeper in- or exhalations, the lung moves downward or upward by about one intercostal space.

On the whole, the left lung sits slightly lower because the liver displaces the lung cranially on the right.

Location of the Fissures

Left Oblique Fissure
This starts in the back near the fourth costovertebral joint and, after a diagonal course around the chest, ends anteriorly in the vicinity of the sixth sternochondral joint.

Anteriorly it is closely connected to ribs 5 and 6, posteriorly to ribs 4 and 5.

Right Oblique Fissure
This starts posteriorly near the third costovertebral joint and ends anteriorly in the vicinity of rib 6.

Anteriorly, it is closely connected to rib 6, posteriorly to ribs 3–6.

Horizontal Fissure of the Right Lung
This originates posteriorly in the oblique fissure below the scapula at the level of rib 4/5 and ends anteriorly slightly below the third sternochondral joint. This joint and rib 4 are located in close proximity to the fissure.

Topographic Relationships

- ribs 1–12, depending on respiratory position
- clavicle
- sternum
- subclavian artery and vein
- phrenic nerve
- pericardiacophrenic artery and vein
- vagus nerve
- recurrent laryngeal nerve
- trachea
- main bronchi
- pulmonary artery and veins
- aorta (left)
- esophagus (right)
- heart (more on the left than on the right)
- diaphragm
- azygos vein
- hemiazygos vein

Attachments/Suspensions

The adhesive force caused by the vacuum in the pleural cavity ensures that the lung does not contract toward the hilum as the result of its own elasticity.

The parietal pleura is firmly attached to the inside of the chest: fascial attachments to the sternum and ribs are found along its entire course. The pleura is also attached solidly to the diaphragm. Toward the mediastinum, it covers the neighboring organs without establishing a firm tie.

At the hilum of the lung caudally, the pulmonary ligament is formed as a fold of the parietal pleura. This ligament is attached to the diaphragm.

At the pleural dome, we find suspensory ligaments that connect the pleura to the first rib and the vertebrae C6–T1:
- costopleural ligament
- transverse pleural ligament
- vertebropleural ligament

Circulation

The pulmonary artery and vein, the vasa publica (i.e., the vessels in charge of gas exchange), branch out from the bronchial tree to reach the capillaries that form a mesh around the alveoli.

The vasa privata (i.e., the vessels that supply the lung tissue itself with oxygen and nutrients) originate as follows.

Arterial

Bronchial branches
- thoracic aorta for the left lung
- third and fourth intercostal arteries for the right lung

Venous

Bronchial veins. They run into the pulmonary veins or into the azygos and hemiazygos veins.

Innervation

Sympathetic Nervous System from T1–T2 to T5–T6
The fibers run to the pulmonary plexus and then on along the bronchial tree into the periphery of the lung.

Parasympathetic Nervous System
Vagus nerve.

Organ Clock

Maximal time: 3–5 a.m.
Minimal time: 3–5 p.m.

Organ–Tooth Interrelationship

For basic information, see page 34.

- Second back tooth in the upper jaw on the left for the left lung
- Second molar in the lower jaw on the left for the left lung
- Second molar in the lower jaw on the right for the right lung
- Second back tooth in the upper jaw on the right for the right lung

■ Anatomy of the Mediastinum

The term "mediastinum" refers to the space in the chest that is bordered as follows.

Anterior. Sternum.

Posterior. Spinal column.

Cranial. Upper thoracic aperture.

Caudal. Diaphragm.

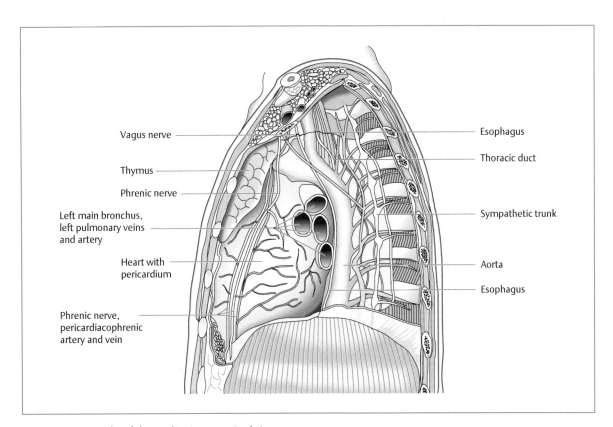

Fig. 17.5 Topography of the mediastinum: sagittal view.

Lateral. Both halves of the lung.

In this space, we find a large number of important structures that are essential for the vitality of the entire body:

- heart with pericardium
- the major arteries and veins of the body:
  - aorta
  - pulmonary artery
  - SVC
  - pulmonary veins
- esophagus
- trachea
- main bronchi
- vagus nerve
- phrenic nerve
- sympathetic trunk
- thymus
- azygos vein
- hemiazygos vein
- thoracic duct

These organs and circulatory structures are linked to each other by connective tissue. This ensures good fixation in the mediastinum. However, sufficient mobility must be present to follow the movements of the torso, arm, and head and neck, e.g., the esophagus and other organs

must be able to stretch in a craniocaudal direction during a neck extension.

Another factor that requires mobility is the expansion of the lung and the movements caused by diaphragmatic breathing. The mediastinum thus experiences alternating pushing and pulling.

Lastly, heartbeats, in the sense of oscillations, also have an impact on the mediastinal structures.

Thus we can see that continuous, even if partly only minor, movements in this apparently motionless space affect the organs of the mediastinum. This fact is particularly significant for the blood flow back into the heart, which is influenced by the suction effect of respiration, and for the nerve structures that are stimulated in the osteopathic sense by this constant movement.

The mediastinum is tied into the fascial system of the "central tendon." It constitutes the thoracic aspect of a fascial pull that reaches from the base of the skull down to the lesser pelvis. As a result, we can see fascial structural adaptations in the mediastinum that could lead to symptoms in the thorax but have their cause in a different location in the body.

As a result of the vital importance of the mediastinal structures, abnormal fascial pulls can lead to significant functional changes. Here, we might consider the vagus innervation or the clinical picture of a hiatus hernia.

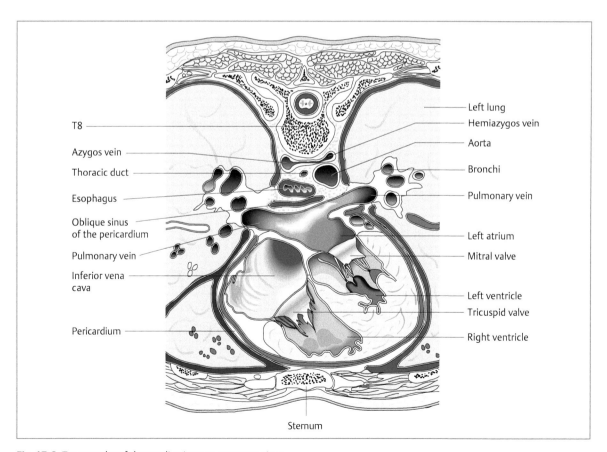

Fig. 17.6 Topography of the mediastinum: transverse view.

Movement Physiology

Respiration is the motor for the regular movement of the thorax. An average of 12–14 breaths/min require the chest to expand and contract rhythmically in its sagittal and transverse diameters.

In biomechanical terms, we distinguish between two movement directions of the ribs: the rotational axis of the upper ribs that runs through the costotransverse and costovertebral joints lies almost parallel to the frontal plane—during inhalation, the result is mainly an expansion of the sagittal diameter of the chest.

The rotational axis of the lower ribs lies almost in the sagittal plane. By raising the ribs during inhalation, the result is thus primarily an enlargement of the transverse diameter of the thorax.

The central ribs have a movement axis that forms a 45° angle to the sagittal plane. Inhalations here lead to an expansion in the sagittal and transverse diameters.

In the sternum, the movement of the ribs causes a rise cranially and an increase in the distance to the spinal column—the sternum moves anteriorly and superiorly during inhalation. Movements therefore occur in both the sternocostal and the chondrocostal joints.

In the chondrocostal junction, the rib cartilages experience a torsion that is of great significance for the elastic and passive return of the thorax from the inhalatory position to the respiratory rest position.

Inhalation is a process that is directed by respiratory muscles: easy respiration involves the diaphragm and the scalene and intercartilaginous muscles. These extend—as described above—the chest in its sagittal and transverse diameters; the diaphragm increases the thorax diameter caudally and raises the lower ribs.

The contraction of the diaphragm causes a movement caudally while pushing the abdominal organs inferiorly and anteriorly. The movement anteriorly results from the soft abdominal wall, which does not provide active resistance against the displacement of the abdominal organs during inhalation.

In easy respiration, exhalation is a passive process, directed by the elastic restorative force of the thorax.

In deep inhalations, additional muscles assist in the expansion of the thorax. These accessory inhalatory muscles include the:
- external intercostals
- serratus posterior superior
- serratus anterior
- greater pectoral
- smaller pectoral
- sternocleidomastoid
- erector muscle of the spine

Deep inhalations cause an extension in the spinal column, as a result of which the extensors of the spinal column can also be included indirectly among the inspiratory muscles.

Forced exhalations likewise involve further accessory expirators:
- abdominal muscles (internal and external oblique, rectus abdominis, transversus abdominis)
- internal intercostal muscle
- subcostal muscle
- transversus thoracis
- serratus posterior superior
- latissimus dorsi

Physiology

■ Physiology of the Heart

Here, we describe the mechanical heart action of the left heart. The same processes take place in the right heart.

Systole

Contraction Phase

- ventricle is filled with blood
- phase starts when the contraction of the ventricle starts

As a result of the contraction of the ventricle, intraventricular pressure rises. When this pressure is greater than the pressure in the atrium, the AV valves close (the semilunar valves are still closed). Tendinous fibers and papillary muscles prevent the AV valves from blowing through into the atrium. The surfaces of the individual flaps are greater than the opening to be closed. By broadly juxtaposing the edges of the flaps, closure of the valve is ensured even when the ventricular size changes. In the ventricle, no change in volume occurs, but only a reshaping of the ventricle into the form of a ball (= isovolumetric contraction). All muscle fibers change their length actively or passively.

Duration of this phase: 60 ms when the body is at rest.

Ejection Phase

This phase starts when the pressure in the left ventricle is greater than the diastolic pressure in the aorta (80 mmHg). The semilunar valves open and pressure continues to rise until it reaches the systolic blood pressure value (approximately 120–130 mmHg). Finally, the ventricular contraction is released and the pressure drops back down. When the pressure is lower than the aortic pressure, the semilunar valve closes and systole is thereby concluded.

During rest, approximately half the contents of the ventricle (130 mL) is ejected (= stroke volume).

Diastole

Relaxation Phase

For approximately 50 ms, all valves are closed. Ventricular pressure drops to almost 0 mmHg—when it falls below atrial pressure (2–4 mmHg), the AV valves open.

Fill Phase

The ventricle fills up in a quick passive phase (see below), caused by the atrial contraction taking place in this phase. With normal heart frequency, the filling of the ventricles is almost completed by the time of the atrial contraction—it receives 8% additional filling by it.

The rapid fill phase of the heart begins during the ejection phase. As we have seen above, blood is pressed out of the ventricle. At the same time, blood is also sucked into the atrium.

The reason for this is that, via the pericardium, the heart is firmly attached to the diaphragm—the apex of the heart is a punctum fixum. The atria are fixed by the vessels and hence also serve as a punctum fixum. The level of the valves is the punctum mobile.

Ventricular contraction moves the heart valves in the direction of the apex. The slackened atria are stretched, which creates suction on the supply vessels of the atria; they fill with blood.

As the ventricular muscles slacken, the valves return to their starting position and the AV valves open. As an inert mass, the atrial blood remains in the same place and the ventricle slides on top of this blood; the rapid passive filling of the ventricle results. This mechanism becomes especially important in heightened frequency with shortened diastole.

Heart Sounds

First Sound = Sound of Contraction
- at the start of systole
- The isovolumetric contraction of the ventricles causes the ventricles and AV valves to vibrate. This creates a sound.

Second Sound = Valve Sound
- at the start of diastole
- The closure of the semilunar valves creates the second heart sound.

Third Sound
Sudden jerk of the ventricular wall caused by blood rushing in during the fill phase of the heart—audible in children.

Fourth Sound
Contraction of the atria—at the end of the P wave in the ECG; physiological in youth, but in adults a sign of increased atrial strain.

Dynamics of the Heart—Adaptation to Changing Strains

The venous backflow into the heart is not constant. When lying down, for example, it is greater than when standing up, due to the effects of gravity. Blood pressure varies almost by the minute. The heart must be able to respond to these constant changes in inflow in such a way that a steady bloodstream without blockages is guaranteed. The two potential disturbances in the continuous blood flow are pressure overload and volume overload.

Acute Volume Overload

For example, infusion or valvular insufficiency.

An increase in end-diastolic filling of the heart causes a greater stroke volume due to self-regulation. This is known as the Frank–Starling law of the heart.

Acute Pressure Overload

For example, rise in blood pressure or valvular stenosis.

The ventricle has to work against increased pressure, and the adaptation occurs in steps:
1. The stroke volume declines because the ventricle is not strong enough to eject the same volume of blood against the elevated pressure.
2. As a result, the rest volume increases.
3. The Frank–Starling mechanism comes into play.

In chronic pressure or volume overload, the heart hypertrophies up to approximately 500 g. As a result of the end-arterial supply of the heart, cardiac insufficiency is a threat.

Energetics of the Heart

The heart operates exclusively under aerobic conditions; similar to the skeletal muscle, it is unable to work without oxygen. During rest, it consumes approximately 10% of the total oxygen consumption in the body and during physical activity up to 40%.

The heart uses up 75% of the oxygen in the coronary arteries during rest. An increased oxygen demand can thus be met only by means of increased circulation.

The coronary arteries fill during diastole; the coronary sinus is squeezed during systole.

The heart processes glucose, free fatty acids, and lactate.

■ Physiology of the Lung

Pulmonary Circulation
In the pulmonary circulation, there are regional differences depending on the position of the body: when standing, the basal parts of the lung are better supplied with blood than the apex of the lung. In contrast, however, the

apex of the lung is ventilated better: The partial pressure of oxygen in the apex of the lung is 114 mmHg, but at the base only 92 mmHg.

Euler–Liljestrand Mechanism

Low partial pressure of oxygen (a measure of the oxygen content in the air) in an alveolar region results in a contraction of the arterioles in this segment. As a result, circulation is reduced in badly ventilated areas of the lung, but blood flow to the well-ventilated areas increases.

If this mechanism causes larger sections of the lung to be taken out of circulation, it can lead to increased resistance in the pulmonary circulation with a greater strain on the right heart. Spinal column deformations such as severe scoliosis can be a cause of this pathology because of reduced chest mobility.

Respiratory Regulation

Respiratory regulation takes place mainly by chemical control of the carbon dioxide and oxygen content of the blood as well as by measuring the pH level.

The carbon dioxide level is therefore the key driving force for respiration: if this value rises in the blood, increased respiration results, to exhale the carbon dioxide. A drop of the pH value to <7.4 has the same effect. The receptors for both of these values are located primarily in the medulla oblongata, where we can also find the respiratory center.

The oxygen level is measured in the arch of the aorta and the carotid sinus, and is processed in the medulla oblongata. If the oxygen level drops to about two-thirds of its normal level, increased respiration ensues. The two other measurements, however, respond much earlier with increased respiration.

Other respiratory stimuli include:
- muscle activity
- warmth or cold
- changes in body temperature
- pain
- epinephrine and progesterone
- drop in blood pressure

Pathologies

Symptoms that Require Medical Clarification

- Signs of angina pectoris
- Sudden decline in performance
- Obstructions in systemic and pulmonary circulation systems
- Dyspnea with in- or expiratory stridor
- Bloody sputum

Coronary Heart Disease

Definition. Constriction of the coronary vessels due to atherosclerotic changes with impaired supply of oxygen to the cardiac muscle.

Causes of atherosclerosis
- familial predisposition
- age
- male sex
- high level of cholesterol (increase in total level and low-density lipoprotein [LDL] level, low high-density lipoprotein [HDL] level)
- elevated triglycerides
- high blood pressure
- diabetes mellitus
- smoking
- lack of exercise
- hypertonicity

Clinical
Angina pectoris:
- Retrosternal pain or feeling of tightness in the chest is precipitated by physical activity, cold, heavy meals and rich foods, or psychological stress, and lasts only a short time.
- Pain can radiate into the arms, shoulders, neck, and lower jaw.
- Pain responds well to GTN spray; episodes also stop after the end of the physical strain.

Heart attack:
- symptoms as in angina pectoris, but they are long-lasting and cannot be affected by medication or rest
- fear
- feeling of weakness
- sweating, nausea, vomiting
- can radiate into the upper abdomen
- tachycardia
- pallor
- cold damp extremities

Obstructive Pulmonary Disease

Definition. Constriction or relocation of the airways.

Causes
- phlegm in the airways
- swelling of the mucous membranes
- spasms of the bronchial muscles
- extrathoracic obstruction
- tumor
- aspiration of foreign bodies

Clinical. Dyspnea with in- or expiratory stridor.

Clinical pictures with an obstruction are, for example:
- bronchial asthma
- bronchitis
- emphysema
- cystic fibrosis
- bronchial tumors
- pseudocroup

Restrictive Pulmonary Disease

Definition. Loss of expandability in the lung, thorax, or diaphragm.

Causes
- lung resection
- lung fibroses
- pleural peel
- bruised pleura
- scoliosis
- respiratory muscle paralysis
- adiposity
- pneumothorax

Clinical. Dyspnea.

Osteopathic Practice

Cardinal Symptoms

- Signs of angina pectoris
- Sudden decline in performance
- Obstructions in the systemic and pulmonary circulation systems
- Dyspnea with inspiratory or expiratory stridor
- Bloody sputum

Typical Dysfunctions

Adhesions/Fixations

Possible causes include:
- fascial cause as manifestation of a secondary adaptation to another dysfunction
- scarification due to surgery
- adhesions in the pleural space, e.g., after infections

Associated Structural Fixations

- T1–T5
- ribs 1–5 on both sides
- clavicle (fascial fixation)
- costosternal joints 1–7 on both sides
- intraosseous lesions in the sternum

Atypical Symptoms

A list of symptoms follows that can be explained by means of osteopathic chains or result from the patient's history (for an explanation of osteopathic chains, see "Atypical Symptoms" in Chapter 5, page 39):
- little thoracic respiratory movement in easy breathing
- greater supraclavicular fossa filled in
- hyperkyphosis of the thoracic spinal column (TSC)
- neck kyphosis (hypomobile cervicothoracic junction)
- history of compression injury in the thorax, e.g., by a seatbelt in a car accident

Indications for Osteopathic Treatment

Loss of Mobility

The volume of air inhaled and exhaled in one breath at rest is approximately 500 mL. Physical exertion leads to heavier breathing with clearly increased respiratory volume. The involvement of the muscles and movement of the ribs and spinal column are clearly greater.

In accordance with the osteopathic principle of economy and the rule that structure and function inform each other, we can deduce that the thorax operates very economically in normal everyday activity at rest: the body has to utilize a minimum of energy to ensure a sufficient oxygen supply. As this form of breathing requires only a minimum of mobility in the thorax, we see a loss of movement in the chest during the course of life—the structure adapts to the required function. This loss of mobility progresses gradually and unnoticed, and syndromes that develop over time are only rarely connected to a limited mobility in the thorax.

Thoracic outlet syndrome, headaches, and humeroscapular periarthritis are just three examples of diverse disorders that require a close examination of mobility in the chest.

Having included the thorax in the fascial system of the "central tendon," we must carefully analyze the posture of the thorax in osteopathic terms to distinguish between cause and effect. Even though the thorax might appear very rigid, it does follow pathologic fascial pulls that lead to postural changes. After surgery in the lower abdomen, e.g., a cesarean section, the surgery-related scarring can cause fascial pulls, which lead the thorax into flexion to relax tension in the scar.

If a postural change persists for a longer period of time, the structure readapts to the function, and independent thorax-related syndromes develop (see above).

The acquired rigidity of the thorax has effects on the organs in the thoracic cavity.

A loss of expandability in the lung ultimately causes strain on the heart, the venous return flow to the heart is reduced as well, and even stimulation of the vegetative nerves by the normal push and pull is reduced.

Contraindications for Osteopathic Treatment

Thoracic techniques can involve a lot of strength and recoil. Accordingly, the contraindications for these techniques are extensive, for example:

- fractures
- osteoporosis
- cardiac irregularities
- heart attack
- unstable angina pectoris
- implanted pacemaker or defibrillator
- tumors
- feverish infections
- recent surgery, e.g., bypass surgery

Notes for Clinical Application

The space enclosed by the two pleural cavities is called the mediastinum. It is noteworthy in this context that no other space in the human body contains such a large number of vital circulatory structures in such a small area. There is no other region in the body where we can see the significance of fascial continuity and movement as clearly as in the mediastinum. A look at embryology can illustrate this.

In an early phase of development (days 24–28), after the yolk sac has been integrated into the embryo as a primary intestinal tube and a first cavity has formed, the mediastinum does not yet exist in its final shape. Nevertheless, developments take place that have great significance for its later functions.

A bodily cavity exists, but is not yet divided into abdominal and thoracic spaces. This cavity is lined with mesodermal tissue that subsequently differentiates to form the peritoneum, pleura, and pericardium/epicardium, with a parietal and visceral lobe each. This means that these three serous membranes share a common embryologic origin and are functionally related! Here, the mesodermal lining of the first cavity of the embryo forms a continuous fascial tissue layer which already in this early stage extends from the future skull area to the future pelvic floor. This fascial cord is referred to as the central tendon.

Peritoneum, pleura, and pericardium/epicardium are integrated into this central tendon as serous membranes. All three respond in the sense of a "fascial contraction" to disturbances of fascial mobility. This is significant because all internal organs are directly or indirectly connected to this serous membrane.

If peritoneum, pleura, or pericardium is impaired in its mobility because it participates in a compensatory mechanism as an aspect of the central tendon, this involvement can therefore affect the organ, to the point of causing a functional disorder with pathophysiologic significance.

How, therefore, are the two separate cavities of the body formed?

The key development here is the migration of the heart from the cervical region into the thorax as a result of the craniocaudal folding of the embryo in the fourth week of development.

The heart is formed in the cervical region and takes its fascial connections with it into the thorax when it moves there. We can regard the extensive ligaments of the heart sac as remnants of this migration (see page 177). They link the pericardium to the diaphragm, sternum, TSC, cervical spinal column, and organs of the thorax, as well as the bronchial tubes, pleura, and esophagus. Just like the pericardium, these ligaments belong to the central tendon. Considering all of these together, they even constitute a very important part of the central fascial cord because this pericardioligamentary complex connects the fascial part of the neck with the diaphragm, and thereby indirectly with the abdomen. Hence it transmits fascial tensions from the skull and neck area across large areas caudally.

The connective tissue or mesoderm cranial to the heart also migrates into the thorax; there, it ends up caudal to the heart and forms the first still incomplete separation layer between the newly formed cavities of the abdomen and thorax. Out of this transverse septum, the future diaphragm develops, as well as the fascial tissue that we call pleuroperitoneal membrane and the striated muscles in the wall of the torso. This means that both the peritoneum and the pleura are involved in the formation of the diaphragm. In this developmental stage, the diaphragm is a fascia and part of the central tendon! Even later, it continues to respond by compensating between the thorax and abdomen and functioning as a fascial structure. Peritoneum and pleura continue to maintain their solid contact with the diaphragm. This is yet another indication that the diaphragm transmits fascial tensions and compensatory patterns from the thoracic cavity to the abdomen.

The division into the lung cavities and mediastinum now takes place in the thoracic cavity: the pericardium develops out of the lining of the thorax, the halves of the lung growing from posterior into the thorax. They also take the lining of the thorax with them as their exterior cover—the pleura is formed. The space that has now formed between the lungs, the diaphragm, the upper thoracic aperture, and the anterior and posterior endothoracic fascia (also the mesodermal lining of the primitive first cavity of the embryo) is referred to as the mediastinum.

Let us emphasize once more the following three points:

1. As the result of its migration from the cervical region into the thorax, the heart and pericardium have extensive fascial contacts in all three planes of the mediastinum.
2. In an early developmental stage, the diaphragm is a fascia; even after development is finalized, it retains the relevant properties.

3. Pleura, pericardium, and peritoneum share a common origin and cooperate in functional terms as part of the central tendon.

Let us now take a closer look at the mediastinum, which can also be regarded as fascia and part of the central tendon. Here, we find a large number of important circulatory structures very close to each other. These are affected by a movement that initially goes unnoticed.

Let us consider the "content" of the mediastinum from anterior to posterior: behind the sternum is the heart sac, which is connected to the sternum via ligaments. On top of the pericardium, roughly in the upper third of the sternum, is the thymus, which performs an important immunologic function during childhood. Lateral to the pericardium are the two phrenic nerves. Further posteriorly, as the next layer behind the pericardium and thymus, the upper third of the mediastinum contains the large vessels that come out of the heart or run into it. Even further behind these, we find the trachea, which divides at the level of T4 into the two main bronchial tubes; these lie against the pericardium.

In the upper third of the mediastinum, further behind the trachea, the esophagus is located, which approximates the pericardium only after the tracheal bifurcation. On the right side, the vagus nerve very quickly approximates the esophagus after entering the thorax; the left vagus nerve must first cross the arch of the aorta before it can also run together with the gullet caudally and across the diaphragm.

Furthest posteriorly, directly before the spinal column, we find the following circulatory structures: azygos and hemiazygos veins, thoracic duct, and, in front of the heads of the ribs, the sympathetic trunk.

Hence we see that the mediastinum is crossed by venous, arterial, lymphatic, sympathetic, and parasympathetic conduits that are important for the abdominal organs. The healthy functioning of these organs therefore depends on the "mediastinum."

How does the mediastinum function?

This space between the sternum and the spinal column, the two halves of the lung, the diaphragm, and the upper thoracic aperture is tightly packed with organs and conduits and in between, as if connecting them all, fascial tissue. As a result, all the structures in the mediastinum depend on each other because they are attached to each other.

Looked at from the outside, little movement seems to take place in this space, but this looks different from an intrathoracic perspective. Each day, we perform approximately 20 000 breaths. This action creates constant pushing and pulling on the mediastinum in a craniocaudal and lateral direction. The sympathetic trunk is therefore moved in a particular fashion by the heads of the ribs.

The heart beats approximately 100 000 times/day. This action again creates permanent vibrations in the mediastinum.

No other region of the body experiences as much movement as the mediastinum, and no other location contains so many important circulatory structures. All these structures apparently need this amount of continuous movement to perform their tasks to the best of their ability.

Osteopathic Tests and Treatment

Test and Treatment of the Ligaments of the Coracoid Process according to Barral

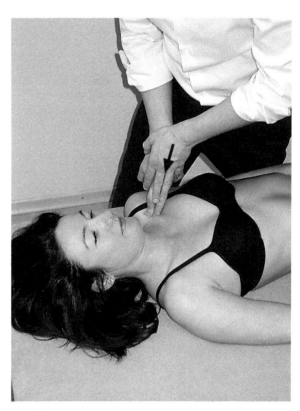

Fig. 17.7

Starting Position
The patient is in the supine position. The practitioner stands on the side to be treated.

Procedure
Palpate the coracoacromial, trapezoid, and conoid ligaments for sensitivity.

To treat, apply frictions or inhibitions to the sensitive areas until the pain has disappeared. Pressure on the sensitive areas should therefore be just strong enough to barely cross the pain threshold. Treatment success can then be evaluated sufficiently.

Test and Treatment of the Costoclavicular Ligament according to Barral

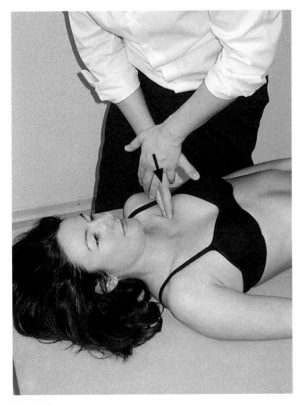

Fig. 17.8

Starting Position
The patient is in the supine position. The practitioner stands on the side to be treated.

Procedure
Palpate the costoclavicular ligament for sensitivity.

To treat, apply frictions or inhibitions to the sensitive areas until the pain has disappeared. Pressure on the sensitive areas should therefore be just strong enough to barely cross the pain threshold. Treatment success can then be evaluated sufficiently.

Compression and Decompression of the Clavicle Along the Longitudinal Axis according to Barral

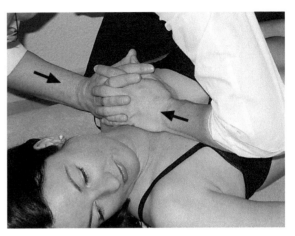

Fig. 17.9

Starting Position
The patient is in the supine position. The practitioner stands on the side to be treated.

Procedure in Compression
With the lateral hand, hold the acromial end of the clavicle between the thenar and hypothenar. With the medial hand, hold the sternal end of the clavicle in the same way. Place the fingers of both hands on top of each other over the clavicle.

Testing Sequence in Compression
Compress the clavicle simultaneously with both hands. Take note of intraosseous and fascial tensions as well as of sensitivity to the compression. In a second step, translate the clavicle laterally and medially.

Treatment in Compression
Translate the clavicle mediolaterally.

For an additional treatment option, you can apply fascial unwinding to the clavicle under compression.

You can conclude treatment with a recoil: increase the compression for one or two breaths during exhalations and maintain during inhalations. When you have reached the greatest possible compression, abruptly release it at the start of the next inhalation.

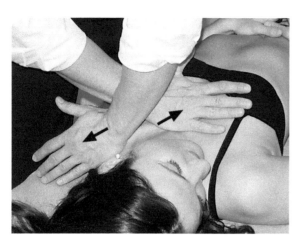

Fig. 17.10

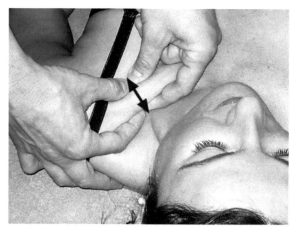

Fig. 17.11

Procedure in Decompression

Position the hands as described above on the sternal and acromial end of the clavicle. Then cross the hands in such a way that the medial hand lies at the acromial end and the lateral hand at the sternal end. The fingers of both hands point away from each other.

Testing Sequence in Decompression

Pull both hands away from each other in the longitudinal direction of the clavicle. Take note of intraosseous and fascial tensions as well as of sensitivity to the decompression.

Treatment in Decompression

Under decompression, palpate the tensions and mobilize by means of intermittent or continuous pulling.

You can conclude treatment with a recoil: increase the decompression for one or two breaths during exhalations and maintain during inhalations. When you have reached the greatest possible decompression, abruptly release it at the start of the next inhalation.

Starting Position

The patient is in the supine position. The practitioner stands on the side to be treated.

Procedure

Place the index fingers of both hands on the posterior side of the clavicle in such a way that it is palpable in its entire length.

Position the thumbs of both hands likewise on the anterior side.

Testing Sequence

Mobilize the clavicle anteriorly and posteriorly over its entire length. Take note of areas of increased fascial tensions and sensitivity.

Treatment

The areas of increased tension can be released by approximating or stretching the tissue. It is also possible to apply a rhythmic mobilization.

Compression and Decompression of the Sternum according to Barral

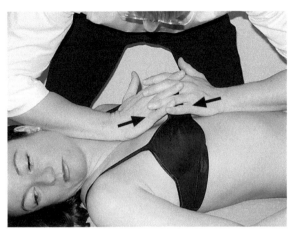

Fig. 17.12

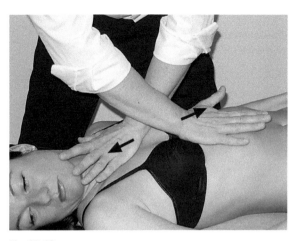

Fig. 17.13

Starting Position in Compression

The patient is in the supine position. The practitioner stands to the side of the patient.

Procedure in Compression

With the cranial hand, hold the cranial end of the sternum between the thenar and hypothenar. With the caudal hand, hold the xiphoid end of the sternum in the same way. Place the fingers of both hands on top of each other on the sternum.

Test in Compression

Compress the sternum simultaneously with both hands. Take note of intraosseous and fascial tensions as well as of sensitivity to the compression.

In a second step, move the sternum cranially and caudally.

Treatment in Compression

Move the sternum in a cranial–caudal direction.

For an additional treatment option, you can apply fascial unwinding to the sternum under compression.

You can conclude treatment with a recoil: increase the compression for one or two breaths during exhalations and maintain during inhalations. When you have reached the greatest possible compression, abruptly release it at the start of the next inhalation.

Procedure in Decompression

Place the hands as described above on the cranial and xiphoid end of the sternum. Then cross the hands and have the fingers of both hands point away from each other.

Test in Decompression

Pull both hands away from each other in the longitudinal direction of the sternum. Take note of intraosseous and fascial tensions as well as of sensitivity to decompression.

Treatment in Decompression

Under decompression, palpate the tensions and mobilize by means of intermittent or continuous pulling.

You can conclude treatment with a recoil: increase the decompression for one or two breaths during exhalations and maintain during inhalations. When you have reached the greatest possible decompression, abruptly release it at the start of the next inhalation.

Mobilization of the Corpomanubrial Junction of the Sternum

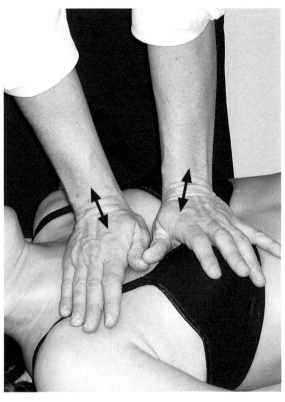

Fig. 17.14

Starting Position
The patient is in the supine position. The practitioner stands to the side of the patient.

Procedure
Place your cranial hand on the manubrium with the thenar at the junction to the sternal body. The caudal hand lies on the sternal body, the thenar on the border to the manubrium. The junction between manubrium and sternal body now lies exactly between the two thenars.

Test
Alternately push the manubrium and sternal body posteriorly. Take note of intraosseous and fascial tensions as well as of sensitivity to mobilization.

Treatment
To mobilize the corpomanubrial junction of the sternum, apply intermittent pressure posteriorly. This technique should be performed with a calm, continuous rhythm until you have released the tensions.

Mobilization of the Corpoxiphoid Junction of the Sternum

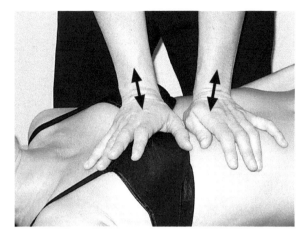

Fig. 17.15

Starting Position
The patient is in the supine position. The practitioner stands to the side of the patient.

Procedure
Place your cranial hand on the sternal body with the thenar at the junction to the xiphoid process. The caudal hand lies on the xiphoid, the thenar on the border to the sternal body. The junction between xiphoid and sternal body now lies exactly between the two thenars.

Test
Alternately push the xiphoid and sternal body posteriorly. Take note of intraosseous and fascial tensions as well as of sensitivity to mobilization.

Treatment
To mobilize the corpoxiphoid junction of the sternum, apply intermittent pressure posteriorly. This technique should be performed with a calm, continuous rhythm until you have released the tensions.

Mobilization of the Sternocostal Joints

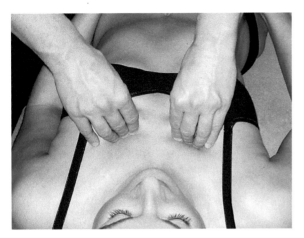

Fig. 17.16

Sternal Lift according to Barral

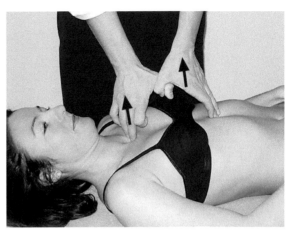

Fig. 17.17

Starting Position

The patient is in the supine position. The practitioner stands to the side of the patient.

Procedure

Grasp the ribs near the sternum between index finger and thumb.

Test

Push the ribs cranially, caudally, and posteriorly. Take note of intraosseous and fascial tensions as well as of sensitivity to the mobilization.

Treatment

The mobilization craniocaudally and posteriorly is applied in a simultaneous movement of both hands in opposite directions, similar to pushing bike pedals when cycling. Apply the mobilization until the tensions are released.

Starting Position

The patient is in the supine position. The practitioner stands to the side of the patient.

Procedure

With the middle finger of the cranial hand, make contact with the sternum in the jugular fossa. The caudal hand holds the tip of the sternum with two fingers on both sides of the xiphoid process. Interlock the thumbs of both hands on top of the sternum, so that you create a pinch grip on the sternum. This grip must be applied gently on both ends of the sternum.

Treatment

Both hands pull anteriorly as if they wanted to pull the sternum out of the thorax. Hold this position for up to 2 min, but in any case long enough to achieve fascial release.

This technique presents a good option for influencing the fascia of the mediastinum.

Mobilization of the Subclavius according to Barral

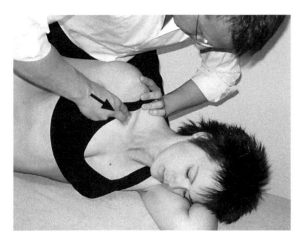

Fig. 17.18

Starting Position
The patient is in the lateral position. The practitioner stands behind the patient.

Procedure
With your cranial hand, hold the patient's shoulder, while working your way into the area below the clavicle with the thumb or one or two fingers of the caudal hand.

Test
Test the subclavius for tensions and sensitivity with the caudal hand.

Treatment
With the caudal hand, fixate the subclavius and remain immobile. With the cranial hand, mobilize the shoulder around the fixed point on the subclavius.

Mobilization of the Transversus Thoracis according to Barral

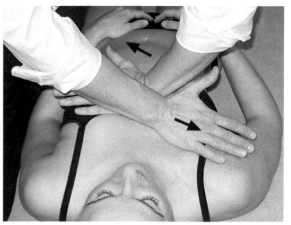

Fig. 17.19

Starting Position
The patient is in the supine position. The practitioner stands to the side of the patient.

Procedure
Imagine the transversus thoracis as an upside-down Christmas tree. Place your caudal hand on the lower third of the sternum and the cranial hand across the other hand, contralateral to the costochondral junction on the ribs (on the left, ribs 2–5; on the right, ribs 3–6).

Treatment
Pull both hands with some pressure away from each other and release with a recoil. Repeat three or four times on each rib attached to the muscle.

Mobilization of the Clavipectoral Fascia according to Barral

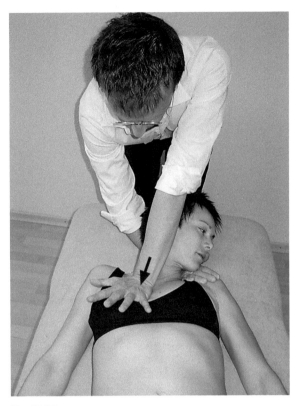

Fig. 17.20

Starting Position
The patient is in the supine position. The practitioner stands at the head of the table.

Procedure
Ask the patient to lift the head and turn it to the left. Now slide your right arm under the head of the patient and take hold of the left shoulder from anterior. Ask the patient to rest his or her head on your lower arm.

Place your left hand with the thenar under the clavicle, fingers pointing in a caudal–lateral direction.

Treatment
Ask the patient to inhale deeply. During the following exhalation, press the left hand in a caudal–lateral and slightly posterior direction. During the next inhalation, maintain the pressure, then increase it again during the exhalation. Repeat this procedure three or four times.

Then abruptly release the pressure at the start of a new inhalation.

Mobilization of the Greater Supraclavicular Fossa

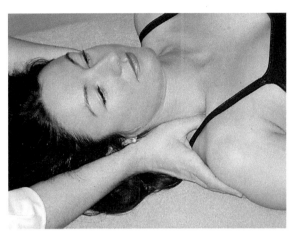

Fig. 17.21

Starting Position
The patient is in the supine position. The practitioner stands at the head of the table.

Test
Place the thumbs of both hands in the greater supraclavicular fossa (GSF). Then test for fascial tension and sensitivity with symmetric pressure caudally.

Treatment
With the thumbs or fingers, apply inhibitions or frictions in the GSF at places with high fascial tension or sensitivity until you have normalized the state of the tissue.

Pectoral Lift according to Barral

Mobilization of the Mediastinum according to Barral

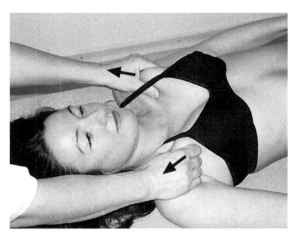

Fig. 17.22

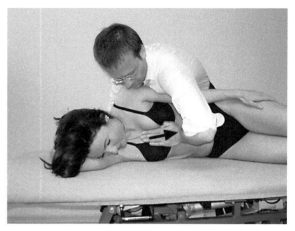

Fig. 17.23

Starting Position

The patient is in the supine position. The practitioner stands at the head of the table.

Treatment

With a pinch grip, grasp the pectoralis major and minor on both sides with your hands. With a strong grip, pull the tissue cranially and maintain the position reached for up to 2 min.

You will quickly notice an obvious fascial release. If the pull is clearly painful at the start, this pain will disappear after only a short time.

Starting Position

The patient is in the lateral position. The practitioner stands behind the patient.

Procedure

Place your anterior hand with the fingertips pointing cranially on the lower third of the patient's sternum. The posterior hand also lies with the fingertips pointing cranially on the spinal column at the level of the manubrium sterni.

Treatment

With the anterior hand, apply pressure caudally and posteriorly; with the posterior hand, apply pressure cranially and anteriorly. Both hands release pressure simultaneously and abruptly (rebound). Repeat this process 8–10 times.

Then position the hands in such a way that the anterior hand lies on the manubrium and the posterior hand on the spinal column at the height of the lower third of the sternum. Now apply pressure with the anterior hand in a cranial–posterior direction and with the posterior hand in a caudal–anterior direction.

Sternocostal Fascial Release in Prone Position

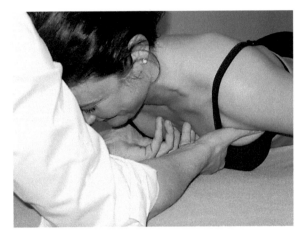

Fig. 17.24

Starting Position
The patient is in the prone position. The practitioner sits at the head of the table.

Procedure
Ask the patient to raise his or her upper body slightly. Place the first to fourth fingers of both hands in the intercostal spaces on both sides in the area of the sternocostal junction. Then ask the patient to lower the upper body back down. Keep your fingers erect.

Variation
You can stay in this position (inhibition) until you feel a fascial release. Alternatively, you can increase the pressure intermittently with different fingers, to reinforce the mobilizing effect.

The fingers can also be positioned on the chondrocostal junction. Treatment is performed in the same way.

Fascial Mobilization on Top of the Coronary Arteries

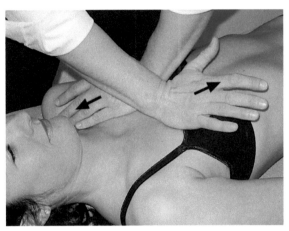

Fig. 17.25

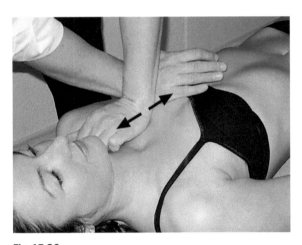

Fig. 17.26

Starting Position
The patient is in the supine position. The practitioner stands on the patient's left side.

Procedure
Cross your hands. Place your left hand on the third sternochondral joint on the left. Place the right hand on the right coronary artery between the third and fourth sternochondral joints on the right. During an exhalation, pull both hands away from each other in a 40° angle to the median line, thereby applying light pressure posteriorly.

For the interventricular branch of the left coronary artery, place the right hand between the third and fourth sternochondral joints on the left. The direction of the pull here is a 20° angle to the median line.

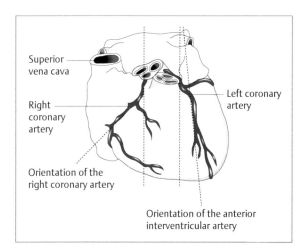

Fig. 17.27 Location of the coronary arteries.

Treatment of the Lung and Pleura

The parietal pleura is tied in its mobility to the thorax. Any technique that mobilizes the thorax at the same time also improves the mobility of the pleura ("external" treatment of the lung). In addition to the techniques described above, you can also utilize stretch positions or clutching grips for treatment.

Techniques from respiratory therapy to maximize ventilation of the lungs can be interpreted as "internal" treatments of the lung. Deeper inhalations and exhalations are also connected to a mobilization of the thorax.

"External" thorax mobilization and "internal" ventilation therapy are a highly effective form of osteopathic lung treatment.

Patients can practice excellent self-mobilizations in this sense by regularly carrying out the Fulford exercises described below.

Circulatory and Reflexive Treatment according to Kuchera

Lymphatic Stimulation

- lymph drainage on thorax and abdomen
- diaphragm techniques

Vegetative Harmonization

Sympathetic nervous system:
- rib raising T1–T6
- inhibiting the paravertebral muscles
- vibrations
- manipulations
- Maitland technique

Parasympathetic nervous system:
Stimulation of the vagus nerve by:
- craniosacral therapy
- laryngeal techniques
- thoracic techniques (recoil)

Reflex Point Treatment according to Chapman

Location—Heart

Anterior. Intercostal space between the second and third ribs, near the sternum (on both sides).

Posterior. Between the two transverse processes of T2 and T3, halfway between the spinous process and the tip of the transverse process (on both sides).

Location—Bronchial Tubes

Anterior. Intercostal space between the second and third ribs, near the sternum (on both sides).

Posterior. On T2, halfway between the spinous process and the end of the transverse process, toward the cranial end of the vertebra (on both sides).

Location—Upper Lung

Anterior. Intercostal space between the third and fourth ribs, near the sternum (on both sides).

Posterior. Between the two transverse processes of T3 and T4, halfway between the spinous process and the tip of the transverse process (on both sides).

Location—Lower Lung

Anterior. Intercostal space between the fourth and fifth ribs, near the sternum (on both sides).

Posterior. Between the two transverse processes of T4 and T5, halfway between the spinous process and the tip of the transverse process (on both sides).

Treatment Principle

Make contact with the reflex point. For this purpose, very gently place a finger on the point and press only lightly. Reflex points are often very sensitive, so it is important to proceed with caution.

The finger remains on the point and treatment is by gentle rotations.

The anterior points are treated first, then the posterior points. Continue with the treatment until you have normalized the sensitivity or consistency of the point.

To conclude, check the anterior points once more. If you fail to notice any change, it is possible that the organ pathology is too great to be influenced quickly via the reflex points, or other dysfunctions are present that must be treated first.

Recommendations for the Patient

Mobility of the Thorax

Deeper breathing requires the thorax to exercise its entire mobility. Physical activity is an effective way to train the maximum mobility of the thorax. Endurance sports are ideally suited for this purpose. They also keep the cardiovascular system and lung function in good condition.

Atherosclerosis Prevention

- physical activity
- no smoking
- reduce weight if overweight

Dietary Recommendations

- Lower cholesterol level and triglycerides.
- Favor polyunsaturated fats over saturated and hydrogenated fats.
- Increase the amount of fiber in the diet.
- Consume garlic, ginger, chili peppers, onions.
- Introduce antioxidants (vitamin A, C, E, etc.) in the form of fruit and vegetables.

The Five Exercises according to Fulford

The following five exercises also aim to improve and maintain mobility in the thorax by means of exercises to be performed on your own. Each exercise should be performed daily for 2 min with gradually deepening breathing that follows the body's own rhythm of breath (as described under "Breathing Exercise").

Exercise 1: Breathing Exercise

Starting Position
Sit up straight on a chair with the feet on the floor, shoulder-width apart and slightly in front of the knees, hands resting on the thighs.

Procedure
Press the tongue against the palate. Now inhale slowly through the nose and exhale through the mouth. To increase airway resistance, the tongue remains up against the palate.

Exercise 2: Stretching the Upper Thorax

Starting Position
Standing with the feet shoulder-width apart.

Procedure
Raise the arms horizontally to shoulder level, one palm pointing up and one pointing down.

Exercise 3: Spinal Column Rotation

Starting Position
Supine position.
   Arms extended horizontally (90° abduction), one hand with the palm facing down, one hand with the palm facing up. The legs are crossed like scissors.

Procedure
Both shoulders should lie on the ground; the crossed leg can lie in a maximum 90° angle to the other leg. After 2 min, switch sides.

Exercise 4: Longitudinal Stretch of the Spinal Column

Starting Position
Sitting on a chair, feet shoulder-width apart.

Procedure
Place the hands on the knees and slide them along the shinbones to the feet. Turn the hands in such a way that the thumbs point outward. Let your head roll gently forward.

Exercise 5: Stretching from the Chest and Abdomen

Starting Position
Standing against a wall.
   Heels, buttocks, shoulders, and back of the head touch the wall.

Procedure
Raise the arms above the head with the backs of the hands to the wall (maximum flexion).

Bibliography

Baenkler HW, Fritze D, Füeßl HS. Duale Reihe Innere Medizin. Stuttgart: Thieme; 2001

Barral JP, Mercier P. Lehrbuch der Viszeralen Osteopathie. Vol.1. 2nd ed. Munich: Urban & Fischer; 2005

Barral JP. Lehrbuch der Viszeralen Osteopathie. Vol.2. 2nd ed. Munich: Urban & Fischer; 2005

Barral JP. The Thorax. Seattle: Eastland Press; 1991

Barral JP. Urogenital Manipulation. Seattle: Eastland Press; 1993

Bouchet A, Cuilleret J. Anatomie. Tome 4. L'abdomen, la région rétro-péritonéale, le petit bassin, le périnée. 2nd ed. Paris: Masson; 2001

Dahmer J. Anamnese und Befund. 10th ed. Stuttgart: Thieme; 2006

Finet G, Williame C. Treating Visceral Dysfunction: An Osteopathic Approach to Understanding and Treating the Abdominal Organs. Portland: Stillness; 2000

Fleischhauer K, eds. Benninghoff Anatomie: Makroskopische und mikroskopische Anatomie des Menschen. Vol.2. 13th/14th ed. Munich: Urban & Schwarzenberg; 1985

Klinke R, Silbernagl S, eds. Lehrbuch der Physiologie. 4th ed. Stuttgart: Thieme; 2005

Knoche H. Lehrbuch der Histologie. Berlin: Springer; 1979

Kobau C. Die Zähne und ihre Wechselbeziehungen zum Organismus. 2nd ed. Self published: Klagenfurt; 2002

Kuchera ML, Kuchera WA. Osteopathic Considerations in Systemic Dysfunction. 2nd ed. Columbus: Greyden; 1994

Lang F. Pathophysiologie—Pathobiochemie. 3rd ed. Stuttgart: Enke; 1987

Langman J. Medizinische Embryologie. 7th ed. Stuttgart: Thieme; 1985

Moore KL. Grundlagen der Medizinischen Embryologie. 2nd ed. Stuttgart: Enke; 1996

Netter FH. Atlas der Anatomie des Menschen. 3rd ed. Stuttgart: Thieme; 2006

Netter FH. Innere Medizin. 1st ed. Stuttgart: Thieme; 2000

Owens C. An Endocrine Interpretation of Chapman's Reflexes. 8th ed. Indianapolis: American Academy of Osteopathy; 1999

Paoletti S. Faszien: Anatomie-Strukturen-Techniken-Spezielle Osteopathie. Munich: Urban & Fischer; 2001

Putz R, Pabst R, eds. Sobotta: Atlas der Anatomie des Menschen. Vol.2. 22nd ed. Munich: Urban & Schwarzenberg; 2006

Richter P, Hebgen E. Trigger Points and Muscle Chains in Osteopathy. Stuttgart–New York: Thieme Publishers; 2009

Rohen JW, Lütjen-Drecoll E. Funktionelle Embryologie. 3rd ed. Stuttgart: Schattauer; 2006

Schmidt RF, Thews G, eds. Physiologie des Menschen. 30th ed. Berlin: Springer; 2007

Schmidt-Matthiesen H, Hepp H, eds. Gynäkologie und Geburtshilfe. 9th ed. Stuttgart: Schattauer; 1998

Schünke M, Schulte E, Schumacher U. Thieme Atlas of Anatomy. General Anatomy and Musculoskeletal System. Stuttgart–New York: Thieme Publishers; 2010

Schünke M, Schulte E, Schumacher U. Thieme Atlas of Anatomy. Neck and Internal Organs. Stuttgart–New York: Thieme Publishers; 2010

Schünke M, Schulte E, Schumacher U. Thieme Atlas of Anatomy. Head and Neuroanatomy. Stuttgart–New York: Thieme Publishers; 2010

Silbernagl S, Despopoulos A. Color Atlas of Physiology. 6th ed. Stuttgart–New York: Thieme Publishers; 2009

Springer Lexikon Medizin. DVD Version 1.3. Berlin: Springer; 2005

Staubesand J, ed. Benninghoff Anatomie: Makroskopische und mikroskopische Anatomie des Menschen. Vol.1. 13th ed. Munich: Urban & Schwarzenberg; 1985

Staubesand J, ed. Sobotta: Atlas der Anatomie des Menschen. Vol.1. 19th ed. Munich: Urban & Schwarzenberg; 1988

Stone C. Visceral and Obstetric Osteopathy. Churchill Livingstone; 2006

Waligora J, Perlemuter L. Anatomie: Enseignement des Centres Hospitalo-Universitaires. 1. Abdomen. Paris: Masson; 1975

Waligora J, Perlemuter L. Anatomie: Enseignement des Centres Hospitalo-Universitaires. 2. Abdomen et petit bassin. Paris: Masson; 1975

Whitaker RH, Borley NR. Instant Anatomy. 2nd ed. Blackwell; 2000

Zenker W, ed. Benninghoff Anatomie: Makroskopische und mikroskopische Anatomie des Menschen. Vol.3. 13th/14th ed. Munich: Urban & Schwarzenberg; 1985

Zimmermann M. Mikronährstoffe in der Medizin. 3rd ed. Heidelberg: Haug; 2003

Index

Page numbers in *italics* refer to illustrations